Fast Facts

D0390738

Prostate cancer

Sixth edition

DISCARD

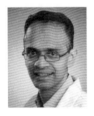

Roger S Kirby MA MD FRCS(Urol) FEBU
Professor of Urology
The Prostate Centre
London, UK

Manish I Patel MBBS MMED FRACS PhD
Senior Lecturer, University of Sydney
Urological Cancer Surgeon
Westmead and Sydney Adventist Hospital
Sydney, Australia

Declaration of Independence
This book is as balanced and as practical as we can make it.
Ideas for improvement are always welcome: feedback@fastfacts.com

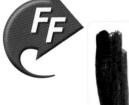

HEALTH PRESS

Fast Facts: Prostate Cancer
First published 1996
Second edition 1998
Third edition 2001
Fourth edition March 2004
Fifth edition May 2008
Sixth edition June 2009

Health Press Limited, Elizabeth House, Queen Street, Abingdon,
Oxford OX14 3LN, UK
Tel: +44 (0)1235 523233
Fax: +44 (0)1235 523238

Book orders can be placed by telephone or via the website.
For regional distributors or to order via the website, please go to:
www.fastfacts.com
For telephone orders, please call 01752 202301 (UK), +44 1752 202301 (Europe),
1 800 247 6553 (USA, toll free), +1 419 281 1802 (Americas) or
+61 (0)2 9698 7755 (Asia–Pacific).

Fast Facts is a trademark of Health Press Limited.

A CIP record for this title is available from the British Library.

ISBN 978-1-905832-57-6

Kirby RS (Roger)
Fast Facts: Prostate Cancer/
Roger S Kirby, Manish I Patel

Medical illustrations by Dee McLean, London, UK.
Typesetting and page layout by Zed, Oxford, UK.
Printed by Latimer Trend & Company Limited, Plymouth, UK.

Text printed with vegetable inks on biodegradable and recyclable
paper manufactured using elemental chlorine free (ECF) wood
pulp from well managed forests.

FSC

Mixed Sources
Product group from well-managed
forests and other controlled sources

Cert no. SGS-COC-005493
www.fsc.org
© 1996 Forest Stewardship Council

Glossary and abbreviations

5α-reductase: the enzyme that converts testosterone to DHT

Antiandrogens: drugs that compete with testosterone or its metabolite DHT for binding to androgen receptors in the prostate

BPH: benign prostatic hyperplasia

Brachytherapy: interstitial radiotherapy

Chemoprevention: the use of drugs to reduce the risk of cancer

Cryoablation: the use of freezing temperatures to destroy tissue

CT: computerized tomography

DES: diethylstilbestrol

DHT: dihydrotestosterone

DRE: digital rectal examination

HDR brachytherapy: high-dose-rate brachytherapy

HIFU: high-intensity focused ultrasound

LHRH: luteinizing hormone-releasing hormone

LHRH agonists: LHRH analogs used to achieve androgen deprivation by inducing chemical castration. They initially stimulate the anterior pituitary resulting in a transient increase in testosterone

LHRH antagonists: pure antagonists that shut off LHRH release obviating the flare phenomenon seen with LHRH agonists

MRI: magnetic resonance imaging

PSA: prostate-specific antigen

TGF: transforming growth factor

TNM: tumor–nodes–metastasis (a staging system for cancer)

TRUS: transrectal ultrasonography

TURP: transurethral resection of the prostate

Introduction

Prostate cancer is the most enigmatic of the common solid malignancies. Second only to lung cancer as a killer of men beyond middle age, it warrants far more attention than it currently receives from governments, researchers and the general public worldwide. One major reason for this continuing neglect is the observation that the majority of men as they age harbor small foci of adenocarcinoma within their prostate that are destined never to become clinically significant. As a consequence, worries about over-diagnosis and over-treatment have surfaced, turning many doctors away from the task of identifying and treating earlier the more aggressive lesions that result in such significant morbidity and mortality.

In fact, the time has come to abandon the prevalent attitude of nihilism about prostate cancer because, potentially, much suffering could be avoided and many lives saved. A number of new ways are becoming available to distinguish the 'tiger' cancers from the 'pussy cats'. Sequential, rather than one-off, prostate-specific antigen (PSA) determinations allow an analysis of PSA kinetics (i.e. change of PSA over time) and this has been shown to be an effective means of identifying so-called high-risk prostate cancers. New molecular markers such as *PCA3*, which is measured from cells in the urine passed immediately after a massage of the gland, offer hope of better specificity and sensitivity than PSA and may avoid the need for prostate biopsy in some men. Moreover, *PCA3* may help distinguish the 'tiger' lesions from the more indolent 'pussy cats'. Other genetically based tests are in the pipeline.

Better staging is also becoming available as enhanced MRI and bone scanning enable us to distinguish with greater certainty those cancers localized to the prostate from those that have already spread to the seminal vesicles, local lymph nodes or to the skeleton itself. These images can be very helpful when deciding which treatment option is most appropriate.

Treatment for prostate cancer itself is also evolving rapidly. For smaller, 'low-risk' tumors, active surveillance with selective delayed intervention is becoming increasingly popular; however, worries persist about the degree of accuracy with which we can detect local or distant progression. The Holy Grail for the management of localized prostate cancer is to eradicate the cancer effectively, while minimizing the collateral damage to adjacent structures such as the neurovascular bundles. New technologies, such as the *da Vinci* robot, that facilitate laparoscopic radical prostatectomy, and low-dose brachytherapy offer this prospect and are rapidly becoming the dominant active treatment options in North America. By contrast, locally advanced prostate cancers are probably best managed by conformal external-beam radiotherapy with pre- and sometimes prolonged post-treatment hormonal ablation.

Once prostate cancer has spread to the lymph nodes or bones, hormonal therapy is usually the first line of treatment and may be effective for many months or years. Eventually, however, hormone resistance develops and second-line treatments need to be considered. Chemotherapy with docetaxel has now been shown to improve survival and several newer therapies, including the endothelin-A-receptor antagonists and the cytochrome P450 inhibitor abiraterone, look promising in this context.

In this sixth edition of *Fast Facts: Prostate Cancer* we have tried to cover all these areas in a concise, informative and evidenced-based fashion. The lives of more and more patients, their families and their supporters, are being touched by prostate cancer; we sincerely hope that this book – with readily accessible and up-to-date information – will be helpful to those who provide their care and treatment.

In most developed and developing countries, prostate cancer is the most commonly diagnosed malignancy affecting men of middle age and beyond, and is second only to lung cancer as a cause of cancer deaths in men. It has been estimated that, in western countries, the lifetime risk of developing microscopic prostate cancer is approximately 30%. At autopsy, the prevalence of microscopic prostate cancer is approximately 80% in men aged 80 years. However, as many of these cancers grow slowly, the risk of developing clinically detectable cancer is about 8%; the lifetime risk of actually dying from prostate cancer is approximately 3%.

Worldwide, there has been a consistent increase in the incidence of clinically significant disease in recent years (Figure 1.1a). Moreover, because prostate cancer is primarily a disease affecting men over the age of 50 years, the worldwide trend towards an aging population means that the number of men diagnosed with prostate cancer is predicted to increase over the next two decades. Mortality from prostate cancer in Europe rose to a peak in 1993, plateaued, and has now started to decrease. Mortality in the USA has recently shown similar trends and has started to decline (Figure 1.1b). The rate of decline has increased significantly in recent years and is now four times faster than the rate in the UK. Some have attributed this drop to the efforts made in North America to detect prostate cancer early, though several other factors such as changes in lifestyle and better treatment may also have contributed.

Risk factors

Despite the high incidence of prostate cancer, relatively little is known about the fundamental causes of the disease. However, a number of risk factors have been established (Table 1.1).

Aging. Age is the greatest factor influencing the development of prostate cancer. Clinical disease is rather rare in men under the age

7

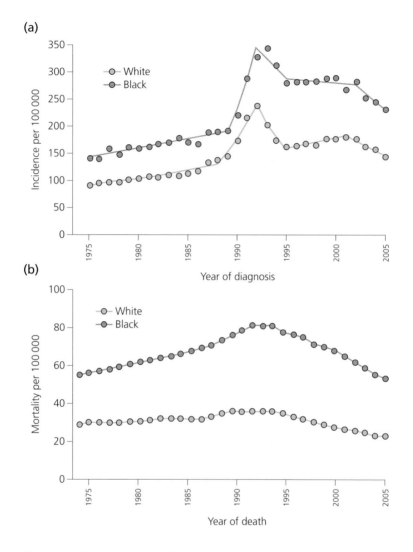

Figure 1.1 (a) The incidence of prostate cancer in the USA from 1975 to 2005. A temporary rise in incidence was noted with the introduction of PSA screening. (b) Mortality from invasive prostate cancer in the USA from 1975 to 2005. Note the consistent decrease in mortality starting from 1993. From Ries LAG et al. *SEER Cancer Statistics Review*, 1975–2005. Bethesda: National Cancer Institute; based on November 2007 SEER data submission, posted to the SEER website, 2008 (http://seer.cancer.gov/csr/1975_2005/).

of 50 years, and the incidence increases markedly in men over 60 years of age (Figure 1.2).

Race. There are marked geographical and ethnic variations in the incidence of clinical prostate cancer. The risk is highest in North America and northern European countries, and lowest in the Far East.

TABLE 1.1

Recognized and possible risk factors for prostate cancer

- Aging
- Race
- Family history
- Hormones
- Genetic polymorphisms

- Obesity
- Western-style diet
- Low exposure to sunlight
- Other environmental factors

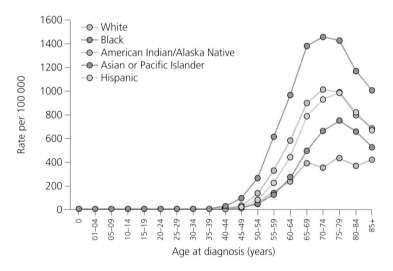

Figure 1.2 Age-specific incidence of prostate cancer by race in the USA from 1977 to 2004 (pooled data). From Ries LAG et al. *SEER Cancer Statistics Review*, 1975-2004. Bethesda: National Cancer Institute: based on November 2006 SEER data submission, posted to the SEER website, 2007 (http://seer.cancer.gov/csr/1975_2004/).

In the USA, the risk is higher in blacks than in whites, and blacks also appear to develop the disease earlier. Chinese and Japanese races show the lowest incidence of prostate cancer, although the prevalence is now increasing within these groups. The incidence of latent disease, however, is similar in all populations studied. In migration studies, the incidence of prostate cancer in men emigrating from a low- to a high-risk area increases to that of the local population within two generations. This suggests that environmental influences such as diet and nutrition may have marked effects on the development of prostate cancer, or on the progression of histological cancer to a clinically detectable cancer.

Family history. Approximately 9% of all cases of prostate cancer have a genetic basis. A number of hereditary prostate cancer (HPC) genes have been localized; the first was on the short arm of chromosome 1. Others have been localized to 1q42.2–43, Xq27–28, p36, 20q13, 16q23 8p22–23, 17p11 and 22q. A number of genetic polymorphisms have also been identified that are associated with the development of prostate cancer. Some centers have reported that genotyping for genetic poly-morphisms can help predict the development of prostate cancer. More research is needed before tests become routinely available. The risk of a man developing prostate cancer if he has a first-degree relative affected is increased approximately 2.5 fold. The relative risks for developing prostate cancer based on family history are given in Table 1.2.

TABLE 1.2

Risk of developing prostate cancer in a man with a family history

Relative affected	Risk (fold increase)
One first-degree relative	2.5
More than one first-degree relative	4.6
Father	2.5
Brother	3.4
Age ≤ 65 years at diagnosis	4.3
Age > 65 years at diagnosis	2.4

Hormones. Testosterone and its more potent metabolite dihydrotestosterone (DHT) are essential for normal prostate growth, and thus may also play a role in the development of prostate cancer (Figure 1.3). Prostate cancer almost never develops in men castrated before puberty, or in men deficient in 5α-reductase (the enzyme, existing in type I and II isoforms, that converts testosterone to DHT). A trial of inhibition of type II 5α-reductase with finasteride has shown that the development of prostate cancer can be reduced by just under 25%, suggesting a role for DHT. However, the incidence of prostate cancer increases with age, while serum testosterone levels decrease. In addition, men diagnosed with prostate cancer have a lower average testosterone level than men of a similar age but without prostate cancer.

Obesity. The suggested link between body mass index and incidence of prostate cancer has been controversial. Early studies showed an increased risk of prostate cancer in obese men, while more recent studies have suggested that obese men actually have lower levels of

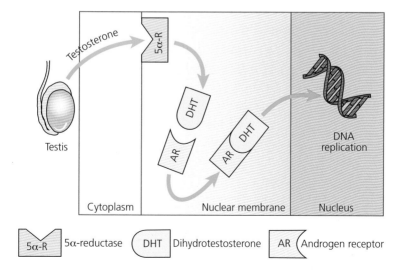

Figure 1.3 Testosterone supports prostate cell function and stimulates cell division.

detected prostate cancer. This may be because levels of prostate-specific antigen (PSA) and androgens are lower in obese men, so fewer obese men may be being biopsied and diagnosed with prostate cancer in the PSA era. There is, however, a clear increase in prostate cancer mortality in men who are obese. The mechanism by which obesity increases the likelihood of death from prostate cancer is not known; it may be through activating procarcinogenic pathways such as the insulin-like growth factor (IGF) axis.

Western diets are high in animal fat, protein, meat and processed carbohydrates, and low in plant foods. A link between dietary fat, saturated fat and meat intake and the development of prostate cancer has been supported by a number of studies. There is also some evidence that α-linoleic acid, an omega-3 polyunsaturated fatty acid, increases prostate cancer risk and the risk of developing advanced prostate cancer. This may be through the development of oxidative stress and subsequent DNA damage or the development of obesity. Omega-3 fatty acids from marine sources are associated with a decreased risk of developing prostate cancer.

Sun exposure and vitamin D. The risk of dying from prostate cancer is geographically related to ultraviolet (UV) light exposure. Vitamin D levels in men with prostate cancer are lower than in men without, and vitamin D levels are determined by dietary intake and conversion in the skin by UV light. The mechanism by which vitamin D levels protect against prostate cancer is not known. Calcitriol (vitamin D) has been used to treat advanced prostate cancer.

Histological features

Most prostate cancers are adenocarcinomas that appear to arise in the peripheral zone of the gland (> 70%) (Figure 1.4). Approximately 5–15% arise in the central zone and the remainder from the transition zone, which is where benign prostatic hyperplasia (BPH) also develops.

Microscopic foci of 'latent' prostate cancer are a common autopsy finding and may appear very early in life; approximately 30% of men over 50 years of age have evidence of latent disease. Because of the very

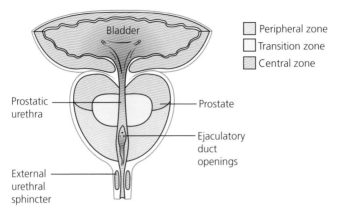

Peripheral zone
Transition zone
Central zone

Bladder

Prostatic urethra

Prostate

Ejaculatory duct openings

External urethral sphincter

Frontal view of normal prostate

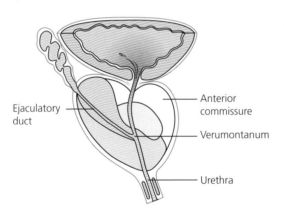

Ejaculatory duct

Anterior commissure

Verumontanum

Urethra

Sagittal view of normal prostate

Figure 1.4 Approximately 70% of prostate cancers arise in the peripheral zone.

slow growth rate of these microscopic tumors, many never progress to clinical disease. Beyond a certain size, however, these lesions progressively dedifferentiate, owing to clonal selection, and become increasingly invasive. A tumor that has a volume greater than 0.5 cm^3 or is anything other than well differentiated is generally regarded as clinically significant.

The Gleason system is the most widely used system for grading prostate cancer (Figure 1.5). It recognizes five levels of increasing aggressiveness.

- Grade 1 tumors consist of small, uniform glands with minimal nuclear changes.
- Grade 2 tumors have medium-sized acini, still separated by stromal tissue, but more closely arranged.
- Grade 3 tumors, the most common finding, show marked variation in glandular size and organization, and generally infiltration of stromal and neighboring tissues.
- Grade 4 tumors show marked cytological atypia with extensive infiltration.
- Grade 5 tumors are characterized by sheets of undifferentiated cancer cells.

Because prostate cancers are often heterogeneous, the numbers of the two most widely represented grades are added together to produce the Gleason score (e.g. 3 + 4). This score (or sum) provides useful prognostic information; Gleason scores above 4 are associated with a progressive risk of more rapid disease progression, increased metastatic potential and decreased survival (Table 1.3). A meta-analysis of patients being managed by active surveillance/watchful waiting (the distinction between the two approaches, as described later, was not clear in the paper), for example, found that the annual rate of developing metastases was 2.1% in patients with Gleason scores of less than 4, compared with 5.4% in patients with scores between 5 and 7, and 13.5% in patients with scores above 7. The chance of relapse after radical prostatectomy has also been shown to be directly proportional to the percentage of Gleason grade 4 and 5 cancer in the specimen. Occasionally, more than two grades are observed in prostatectomy specimens, the least common being known as the tertiary grade. When the tertiary grade has a high score (4 or 5), the patient has a higher risk of progression even if the primary and secondary grades are lower.

One study of 767 men with localized prostate cancer reported a highly significant correlation between the Gleason score and the risk of dying from prostate cancer. Patients with a score of 2–4 had a 4–7% chance of dying within 15 years of diagnosis. In contrast, patients with a score of 8–10 had a 60–87% chance of death from prostate cancer.

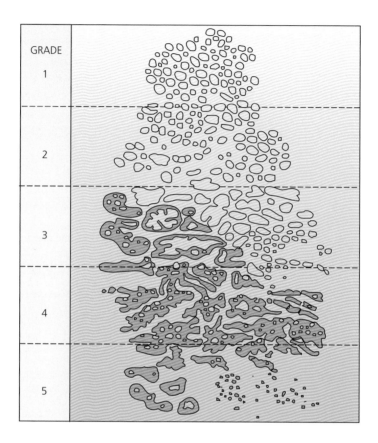

Figure 1.5 The Gleason grading system is based on the extent to which the tumor cells are arranged into recognizably glandular structures. Grade 1 tumors form almost normal glands that are progressively lost through the grades. By grade 5, tumors are characterized by sheets of undifferentiated cancer cells. In individual patients, the prognosis worsens with the progressive loss of glandular differentiation. Because prostate cancers are often heterogeneous in histological pattern, the Gleason score (or sum) is calculated by the summation of the grades of the two predominant areas. Adapted from Gleason DF. The Veterans' Administration Cooperative Urologic Research Group: Histologic grading and clinical staging of prostatic carcinoma. In: Tannenbaum M, ed. *Urologic Pathology: The Prostate.* Philadelphia: Lea and Febiger, 1977:171–98.

TABLE 1.3

The Gleason score*

Gleason score	Histological characteristics	10-year likelihood of local progression (%)
2–6	Well differentiated	25
7	Moderately differentiated	50
8–10	Poorly differentiated	75

*The Gleason score is the sum of the two most prominent grades.

Patterns of disease spread

Prostate cancer can be classified according to the spread of the disease by the tumor–nodes–metastasis (TNM) system (Table 1.4). The tumor stage (T1–T4) describes the pathological development of the tumor.

- T1 represents 'incidental' status, in which the tumor is discovered after transurethral resection of the prostate (TURP) or more commonly by PSA testing, and is not detectable by palpation or ultrasonography.

TABLE 1.4

The TNM classification of prostate cancer (2002)

Primary tumor

Tx   Primary tumor cannot be assessed

T0   No evidence of primary tumor

T1   Clinically inapparent tumor not palpable or visible by imaging

    T1a   Tumor incidental; histological finding in 5% or less of tissue resected

    T1b   Tumor incidental; histological finding in more than 5% of tissue resected

    T1c   Tumor identified by needle biopsy (e.g. because of elevated PSA)

(CONTINUED)

TABLE 1.4 (CONTINUED)

T2 Tumor confined within the prostate*

    T2a Tumor involves 50% or less of one lobe

    T2b Tumor involves more than 50% of one lobe but not both lobes

    T2c Tumor involves both lobes

T3 Tumor extends through the prostatic capsule[†]

    T3a Extracapsular extension (unilateral or bilateral)

    T3b Tumor invades seminal vesicle(s)

T4 Tumor is fixed or invades adjacent structures other than seminal vesicles: bladder neck, external sphincter, rectum, levator muscles and/or pelvic wall

Regional lymph nodes

Nx Regional lymph nodes cannot be assessed

N0 No regional lymph node metastasis

N1 Regional lymph node metastasis

Distant metastasis[‡]

Mx Distant metastasis cannot be assessed

M0 No distant metastasis

M1 Distant metastasis

    M1a Non-regional lymph node(s)

    M1b Bone(s)

    M1c Other site(s)

*Tumor found in one or both lobes by needle biopsy, but not palpable or visible by imaging, is classified as T1c.
[†]Invasion into the prostatic apex or into (but not beyond) the prostatic capsule is not classified as T3, but as T2.
[‡]When more than one site of metastasis is present, the most advanced category should be used.

- T2 and T3 are intermediate stages.
- T4 represents advanced disease, in which the tumor invades neighboring organs (Figure 1.6).

The nodal stages (N0–N1) and metastatic stages (M0–M1c) reflect the clinical progression of the disease. Metastases are most common in the lymph nodes (N1) and bones (M1); the lungs and other soft tissues are less commonly involved.

Currently, it is not possible to distinguish unambiguously between those tumors that will remain latent throughout the patient's life and those that will definitely progress to clinical disease. Studies of incidental carcinomas diagnosed after TURP suggest that the median time to

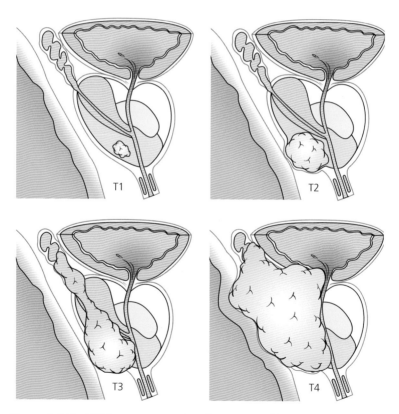

Figure 1.6 The TNM system recognizes four stages of local tumor growth, from T1 (incidental) to T4 (invasion of neighboring organs).

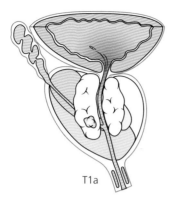
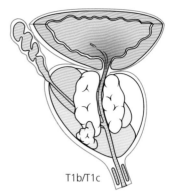

T1a

T1b/T1c

Figure 1.7 Incidental carcinoma of the prostate is unsuspected cancer diagnosed at TURP. T1a cancers are small, well-differentiated lesions involving less than 5% of resected tissue. T1b cancers are larger, involve more than 5% of the resected chippings and are less well differentiated. T1c cancers detected by PSA testing are usually greater than 0.5 cm^3 in volume and moderately well differentiated.

progression for T1b (high-volume, moderately or poorly differentiated) tumors is 4.75 years, compared with 13.5 years for T1a (low-volume, well-differentiated) tumors (Figure 1.7). Thus, elderly men with T1a tumors are more appropriately managed by active surveillance alone, while younger men with T1b disease may be considered for more aggressive, potentially curative therapy.

Key points – epidemiology and pathophysiology

- Prostate cancer is soon likely to become the most common cause of cancer death in men.
- Age is the greatest risk factor, but race, family history, western-style diet and obesity also have an impact.
- Most prostate cancers are adenocarcinomas arising in the peripheral zone.
- Prostate cancers are graded according to the Gleason system.

Key references

Albertsen PC, Hanley JA, Fine J. 20-year outcomes following conservative management of clinically localized prostate cancer. *JAMA* 2005;293:2095–2101.

Baillargeon J, Pollock BH, Kristal AR et al. The association of body mass index and prostate-specific antigen in a population-based study. *Cancer* 2005;103:1092–5.

Calle EE, Rodriguez C, Walker-Thurmond K, Thun MJ. Overweight, obesity, and mortality from cancer in a prospectively studied cohort of U.S. adults. *N Engl J Med* 2003;348:1625–38.

Chen C. Risk of prostate cancer in relation to polymorphisms of metabolic genes. *Epidemiol Rev* 2001;23:30–5.

Engeland A, Tretli S, Bjorge T. Height, body mass index, and prostate cancer: a follow-up of 950000 Norwegian men. *Br J Cancer* 2003;89:1237–42.

Giovannucci E, Liu Y, Platz EA, Stampfer MJ, Willett WC. Risk factors for prostate cancer incidence and progression in the health professionals follow-up study. *Int J Cancer* 2007;121:1571–8.

Johns LE, Houlston RS. A systematic review and meta-analysis of familial prostate cancer risk. *BJU Int* 2003; 91:789–94.

Langeberg WJ, Isaacs WB, Stanford JL. Genetic etiology of hereditary prostate cancer. *Front Biosci* 2007;12:4101–10.

Leitzmann MF, Stampfer MJ, Michaud DS et al. Dietary intake of n-3 and n-6 fatty acids and the risk of prostate cancer. *Am J Clin Nutr* 2004;80:204–16.

Levi F, Lucchini F, Negri E et al. Leveling of prostate cancer mortality in Western Europe. *Prostate* 2004;60:46–52.

Lu-Yao GL, Greenberg ER. Changes in prostate cancer incidence and treatment in USA. *Lancet* 1994; 343:251–4.

Montironi R, Mazzucchelli R, Scarpelli M. Precancerous lesions and conditions of the prostate: from morphological and biological characterization to chemoprevention. *Ann N Y Acad Sci* 2002;963:169–84.

Moyad MA. Lifestyle/dietary supplement partial androgen suppression and/or estrogen manipulation. A novel PSA reducer and preventive/treatment option for prostate cancer? *Urol Clin North Am* 2002;29:115–24.

Nelson MA, Reid M, Duffield-Lillico AJ, Marshall JR. Prostate cancer and selenium. *Urol Clin North Am* 2002;29:67–70.

Nelson PS, Brawer MK. Chemoprevention of prostatic carcinoma. *Urology Int* 1997;4:7–9.

Parker SL, Tong T, Bolden S, Wingo PA. Cancer statistics, 1996. *CA Cancer J Clin* 1996;46:5–27.

Porter MP, Stanford JL. Obesity and the risk of prostate cancer. *Prostate* 2005;62:316–21.

Quinn M, Babb P. Patterns and trends in prostate cancer incidence, survival, prevalence and mortality. Part I: international comparisons. *BJU Int* 2002;90:162–73.

Roberts R, Jacobsen S, Kalusic SK et al. Recent declines in prostate cancer incidence and mortality. *J Urol* 1998;159:123A.

Ross RK, Bernstain L, Lobo RA et al. 5-alpha-reductase activity and risk of prostate cancer among Japanese and US white and black males. *Lancet* 1992;339:887–9.

Schwartz GG. Vitamin D and intervention trials in prostate cancer: from theory to therapy. *Ann Epidemiol* 2008; Epub ahead of print.

Thompson IM, Goodman PJ, Tangen CM et al. The influence of finasteride on the development of prostate cancer. *N Engl J Med* 2003;349: 215–24.

Zheng SL, Sun J, Wiklund F et al. Cumulative association of five genetic variants with prostate cancer. *N Engl J Med* 2008;358:910–19.

Diet, lifestyle and chemoprevention

Effect on development of prostate cancer

Diet and lifestyle are clearly linked to the development of prostate cancer. In Chapter 1, the effect of hormones, obesity and a western-

TABLE 2.1

Effects of dietary manipulation to reduce the incidence of prostate cancer

Compound	Source	Maximum suggested effect
Calcium	• Dietary supplements • Dairy products	• Reported to increase risk by up to 70% in some studies
Fish oils	• Oily fish	• Reduction up to approximately 45% from eating oily fish > 3 times/week
Lycopene	• Tomatoes • Watermelon • Pink grapefruit • Guava	• 15–20% reduction, increasing to 25% if > 2 servings of tomato product/week
Saturated fat	• Saturated fats, including red meat and dairy	• 10–30% increase
Selenium	• Grains • Fish • Meat • Poultry • Dairy products	• Approximately 50% reduction with 200 µg daily • Excessive intake can be toxic
Soy/ isoflavonoids	• Soy products	• Up to 70% reduction if > 1 serving of soy milk daily
Vitamin D	• Supplements • Sunlight	• Not established
Vitamin E	• Supplements	• Approximately 30% reduction with 50 mg daily
Zinc	• Dietary supplements	• Not established but concerns that supplements may increase risk

style diet were discussed as risk factors for the development of prostate cancer. A large number of studies have evaluated the effects of dietary manipulation/supplementation or drug treatment to reduce the incidence of prostate cancer. Table 2.1 shows the current evidence for dietary manipulation.

Randomized clinical trials have provided some indication of a protective effect from selenium and vitamin E. A large chemoprevention

Strength of evidence	Comment
• Medium	• Conflicting study results but many also show no increased risk
• Medium	• Omega-3 fatty acids from marine sources thought to offer a protective role
• Medium	• Better effect with cooked or processed tomato products (e.g. tomato sauce)
• Poor	• Associations with total fat, saturated fat, meat and linoleic acid have been reported
• Medium	• Some evidence of effect, particularly in those with low PSA levels and low plasma selenium levels, but results from large randomized controlled trial were disappointing
• Medium	• No strong evidence but lower level evidence consistently supports an effect
• Poor	• No substantial evidence to support an effect
• Medium	• Some suggestion of an effect, but results from large randomized controlled trial were disappointing
• Poor	• Epidemiological and experimental data are conflicting

study (SELECT), designed to determine whether they reduced the likelihood of prostate cancer when used singly or in combination, was ended prematurely because of disappointing results. Cohort studies show that lycopene, which is found in tomatoes, and isoflavonoids from soy products are associated with a decrease in the incidence of prostate cancer. Evidence for other dietary supplements is weak.

Chemoprevention with drugs. The 5α-reductase inhibitor finasteride has been shown to reduce the incidence of prostate cancer by 24.8% compared with placebo over a 7-year period, though at the cost of a small incidence of sexual side effects. Counterbalancing this observation is the finding that the cancers that did occur in the finasteride group tended to be more aggressive in nature than those occurring in the placebo group. The explanation for this is still debated, but it is possibly explained by an artifact of biopsying the smaller prostates that result from the shrinkage effect of finasteride in the active treatment arm of the study.

Another 5α-reductase inhibitor, dutasteride, has been evaluated for its effect on the occurrence of prostate cancer in the so-called REDUCE study (Reduction by Dutasteride of Prostate Cancer Events). Dutasteride resulted in a 23% reduction in prostate cancer risk, mainly by suppressing the well-differentiated cancers, with no increase in Gleason pattern 7 or 8–10 poorly differentiated tumors. It also effectively treated the symptoms arising from benign prostatic enlargement in participants.

Effect on prostate cancer progression

Unfortunately, very few clinical trials have been performed on the effect of diet and lifestyle change on prostate cancer progression. Table 2.2 outlines the current body of evidence. In addition to this, a large number of compounds – many of them herbal – have been tested in the laboratory and show possible promise; these include green tea and other polyphenols, resveratrol from red wine, vitamin D, epilobium and *Serenoa repens* (saw palmetto).

It must be remembered that the major killer in men with or without prostate cancer is cardiovascular disease. To improve mortality in men

TABLE 2.2

Effect of diet and lifestyle on prostate cancer progression

Factor and effect	Comment
Exercise	
No clear evidence but suspected to be of benefit	Performance index is an independent prognostic indicator in clinical trials
Low-fat diet	
Possible reduction in cancer growth	Low level of clinical benefit based on animal and human biomarker studies
Fish oils/omega-3 fatty acids	
Possible reduction in cancer growth	Based on a cohort study and an animal study
Lycopene	
Reasonable evidence of a reduction in PSA and tumor size	2 servings per week associated with 20% risk reduction from cohort and animal studies
Pomegranate juice	
Possible reduction in PSA rise after prostate cancer recurrence	Based on low-level evidence from phase II trials
Soy/isoflavonoids	
Inconclusive evidence of any benefit	In-vitro results favorable but an animal study was not supportive

with prostate cancer, heart-healthy lifestyle choices must be made. These include improving lipid profiles, decreasing obesity, increasing fitness and increasing fish oil intake. Not only will these measures decrease the risk of death from cardiovascular causes, but a healthy diet and regular vigorous exercise may help fight the cancer as well.

Key points – diet, lifestyle and chemoprevention

- In a trial, dutasteride reduced the incidence of prostate cancer by about one-quarter over 4 years, and also treated benign prostatic hyperplasia symptoms.
- Men should be advised/supported to lower lipid profiles, decrease obesity, increase fitness and increase their intake of fish oil as part of a strategy to cut the risk of cardiovascular disease and, possibly, prostate cancer.

Key references

Andriole G. Further analyses from the REDUCE prostate cancer risk reduction trial. *Late-Breaking Abstract 1*. Presented at the American Urological Association (AUA) Annual Meeting, 25–30 April 2009, Chicago, IL, USA.

Brooks JD, Metter EJ, Chan DW et al. Plasma selenium level before diagnosis and the risk of prostate cancer development. *J Urol* 2001;166:2034–8.

Cohen YC, Liu KS, Heyden NL et al. Detection bias due to the effect of finasteride on prostate volume: a modeling approach for analysis of the Prostate Cancer Prevention Trial. *J Natl Cancer Inst* 2007;99;1366–74.

Duffield-Lillico AJ, Dalkin BL, Reid ME et al. Selenium supplementation, baseline plasma selenium status and incidence of prostate cancer: an analysis of the complete treatment period of the Nutritional Prevention of Cancer Trial. *BJU Int* 2003;91:608–12.

Giovannucci E, Liu Y, Platz EA, Stampfer MJ, Willett WC. Risk factors for prostate cancer incidence and progression in the health professionals follow-up study. *Int J Cancer* 2007;121:1571–8.

Gomella L. Chemoprevention using dutasteride: the REDUCE trial. *Curr Opin Urol* 2005;15:29–32.

Lippmani SM, Klein EA, Goodman PJ et al. Effect of selenium and vitamin E on risk of prostate cancer and other cancers: the Selenium and Vitamin E Cancer Prevention Trial (SELECT). *JAMA* 2009;301:39–51.

Lucia MS, Epstein JI, Goodman PJ et al. Finasteride and high-grade prostate cancer in the Prostate Cancer Prevention Trial. *J Natl Cancer Inst* 2007;99:1375–83.

Miller EC, Giovannucci E, Erdman JW Jr et al. Tomato products, lycopene, and prostate cancer risk. *Urol Clin North Am* 2002;29:83–93.

Shepherd BE, Redman MW, Ankerst DP. Does finasteride affect the severity of prostate cancer? A causal sensitivity analysis. *J Am Stat Assoc* 2008;103:1392–1404.

Thompson IM, Chi C, Ankerst DP et al. Effect of finasteride on the sensitivity of PSA for detecting prostate cancer. *J Natl Cancer Inst* 2006;98:1128–33.

Thompson IM, Goodman PJ, Tangen CM et al. The influence of finasteride on the development of prostate cancer. *N Engl J Med* 2003;349:215–24.

Virtamo J, Pietinen P, Huttunen JK et al. Incidence of cancer and mortality following alpha-tocopherol and beta-carotene supplementation: a postintervention follow-up. *JAMA* 2003;290:476–85.

The past decade has seen a significant downward shift in the stage at presentation of prostate cancer in most countries. Historically, most men with significant disease presented with a combination of weight loss, bone pain, lethargy and bladder outflow obstruction attributable to locally advanced or metastatic disease. Increasingly, however, the disease is being diagnosed incidentally by prostate cancer screening in younger, asymptomatic patients, and occasionally as an incidental histological finding following a TURP for benign obstructive symptoms. This earlier presentation of prostate cancer has posed difficult dilemmas concerning management for clinicians and patients, and the increasing life-expectancy of patients (Figure 3.1) underscores the need for effective, evidence-based diagnosis and treatment regimens.

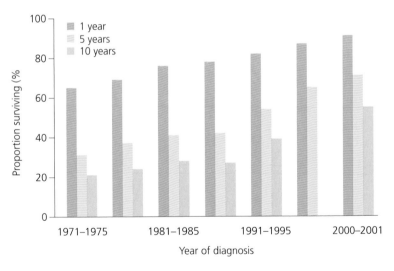

Figure 3.1 Relative survival (%) at 1, 5 and 10 years after diagnosis of prostate cancer in England and Wales (men diagnosed between 1971 and 2001). Note that 10-year data were not available for 1996–2000. Reproduced from Cancer Research UK, http://info.cancerresearchuk.org/cancerstats/types/prostate/survival/

Early detection

In general, the earlier prostate cancer is detected, the better the outlook for the patient in terms of cure or arresting cancer progression. Most patients in whom prostate cancer is suspected are identified on the basis of abnormal findings on digital rectal examination (DRE) or, more commonly now, by raised levels of prostate-specific antigen (PSA). An increasing majority of patients present simply with an isolated increase in PSA.

Digital rectal examination is the simplest, safest and most cost-effective means of detecting prostate cancer, provided that the tumor is posteriorly situated and is sufficiently large to be palpable. The test can be performed with the patient either in the left lateral position or standing and leaning forwards; with either approach only the posterior portion of the gland is palpable (Figure 3.2). In addition to providing information on the size of the prostate, DRE can reveal a number of features that may indicate prostate cancer (Table 3.1). However, only around one-third of suspicious prostatic nodules are actually confirmed as malignant when analyzed histologically after transrectal biopsy (Table 3.2).

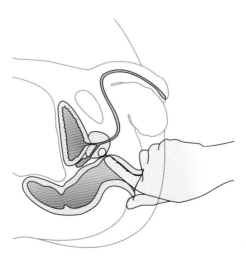

Figure 3.2 DRE is an essential clinical test in the detection and diagnosis of prostate cancer.

TABLE 3.1

DRE findings that may indicate prostate cancer

- A nodule within one lobe of the gland
- Induration of part or all of the prostate
- Asymmetry of the gland
- Lack of mobility due to adhesion to surrounding tissue
- Palpable seminal vesicles

TABLE 3.2

Causes of false-positive diagnoses of prostate cancer on DRE

- Benign prostatic hyperplasia
- Prostatic calculi
- Prostatitis (particularly granulomatous prostatitis)
- Ejaculatory duct abnormalities
- Seminal vesicle abnormalities
- Rectal mucosal polyp or tumor

Prostate-specific antigen is a glycoprotein responsible for liquefying semen. PSA measurement is the most effective single screening test for early detection of prostate cancer; in fact, it can detect more than twice as many prostate cancers as DRE. However, the predictive value is increased further if the measurement is combined, as it always should be, with DRE. PSA determinations may also be useful in staging prostate cancer and evaluating the response to therapy (see Chapter 4).

Approximately 25% of men with PSA levels above the normal range (≥ 4 ng/mL) have prostate cancer, and the risk increases to more than 60% in men with PSA levels above 10 ng/mL (Figure 3.3). Causes of PSA elevation in the absence of prostate cancer are given in Table 3.3. A recent study in prostate cancer prevention, where all men in the placebo group received a biopsy, reported that the incidence of prostate cancer in men with PSA less than 4 ng/mL and normal DRE was high (Table 3.4). The median PSA and 95th percentile values for the 'normal' population

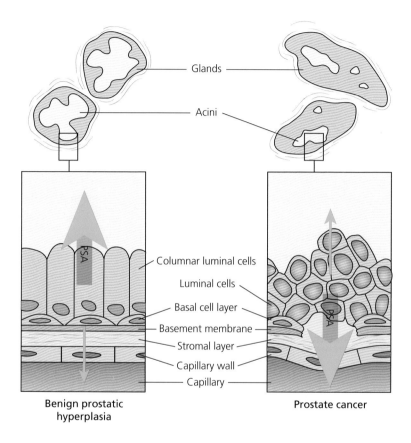

Figure 3.3 Normally, there are significant tissue barriers between the lumen of the prostate gland and the capillary bed. In prostatic diseases, especially cancer, these barriers are compromised, and serum PSA values rise.

TABLE 3.3

Causes of PSA elevation

- Prostate cancer
- BPH
- Prostatitis
- Urinary tract infection
- Perineal or prostatic trauma
- Recent ejaculation
- Bicycle riding

at each age group have been determined and are given in Table 3.5. As shown by the data in Table 3.4, a significant percentage of men with PSA values below the 95th percentile will harbor prostate cancer. There is no clear agreement on the best PSA cut-off at which men should be biopsied. In the past a cut-off of 4.0 ng/mL was used, but it has been shown that a cut-off at 2.5 ng/mL will double the cancer detection rate from 18% to 36% in men younger than 60 years, and will have a minimal negative effect on specificity.

Early results from two large randomized studies have been reported. The larger European study (the European Randomized Study of Screening for Prostate Cancer) randomized men to screening at 4-yearly intervals or no screening. A biopsy was mandated if the PSA was above 3.0 ng/ml or an abnormal DRE was detected. This study reported a 27% reduction in prostate cancer mortality at a median follow-up of

TABLE 3.4

Likelihood of prostate cancer on biopsy in men with normal DRE

PSA value (ng/mL)	Risk of prostate cancer on biopsy (%)
< 0.5	6.6
0.5–1.0	10.1
1.1–2.0	17.0
2.1–3.0	23.9
3.1–4.0	26.9

Source of data: Thompson et al., 2004.

TABLE 3.5

Median and 95th percentile ranges of PSA in a male population

Age range (years)	Median PSA (ng/mL)	95th percentile
40–49	0.7	2.5
50–59	0.9	3.5
60–69	1.3	4.5
70–79	1.8	6.5

9 years. Unfortunately, the number of men needed to treat to save one man from death was 48. In contrast, the smaller US study (the Prostate, Lung, Colorectal, and Ovarian [PLCO] Cancer Screening Trial) did not report a mortality benefit at a shorter follow-up. This trial was also flawed by excessive screening in the control arm.

It is clear that PSA is by no means a perfect test, as many men with mildly elevated PSA values do not have prostate cancer. As a result, several different concepts have been developed over the past few years to improve the clinical value of the test in detecting early prostate cancer. These so-called PSA derivatives include PSA density, PSA velocity, age-specific reference ranges and differential assay of the different molecular forms of serum PSA. All of these have been proposed in an attempt to enhance the utility of PSA with regard to detecting early prostate cancer at a curable stage and to reduce the number of negative transrectal biopsies. In practical terms, only the molecular forms (free:total PSA ratio) and PSA velocity calculation are clinically useful, as they can help the physician and patient decide whether and when to proceed to a transrectal biopsy.

PSA density is calculated by dividing the total PSA by the prostate volume. A PSA density above 0.15 ng/mL has been shown to increase the specificity of the PSA test. This modification does, however, have many potential sources of error, such as volume calculation, assay variability and sampling bias (Figure 3.4).

PSA velocity refers to the rate of PSA change with time, usually over 1 or 2 years, with a minimum of three readings. A velocity above 0.75 ng/mL/year has been used to predict the presence of prostate cancer. More recent studies have shown that the average PSA velocity of men without prostate cancer is 0.03 ng/mL/year, compared with 0.4 ng/mL/year in men ultimately diagnosed with prostate cancer. Most recommend a PSA velocity of 0.35–0.4 ng/mL/year as a threshold to recommend biopsy, even if the PSA is within the normal range. Problems associated with PSA velocity include inaccuracy of velocity calculation over short time periods and too few measurements being made (PSA levels show natural fluctuation).

Age-specific reference ranges are predicated on the fact that the serum PSA concentration increases with age. As a result, the reference

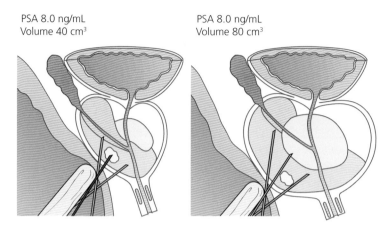

PSA 8.0 ng/mL
Volume 40 cm³

PSA 8.0 ng/mL
Volume 80 cm³

Figure 3.4 Biopsies taken from a larger prostate with a lower PSA density are less likely to sample the cancer than those taken from a smaller prostate with a higher PSA density.

range is corrected for the patient's age (see Table 3.5). This practice increases positive-predictive values from 37% to 42%, but decreases cancer detection when compared with a cut-off of 4.0 ng/mL. Recent studies have shown that age-specific median PSA values may be more useful than age-specific cut-offs, as young patients with a PSA above their age-specific median value but below a biopsy threshold of 2.5 ng/mL have an 8–14-fold increase in the risk of developing prostate cancer. Figure 3.5 shows the problem with using an age-specific cut-off rather than a standard cut-off for all ages – too many cancers are missed in older men (in whom the prevalence is greater).

Molecular forms. PSA exists in the serum in several molecular forms; most of it is bound to protein, but some is unbound or 'free'. Studies show that patients with BPH but not prostate cancer have a higher amount of free PSA, while men with prostate cancer appear to have a greater amount of PSA complexed with α_1-antichymotrypsin. Measuring the concentration of these different molecular forms in the serum is a clinically useful way to distinguish men who have BPH from men with early prostate cancer. The currently accepted cut-off point of free:total PSA is 0.15. Men with ratios below this should be considered for further investigation, including transrectal prostatic biopsy.

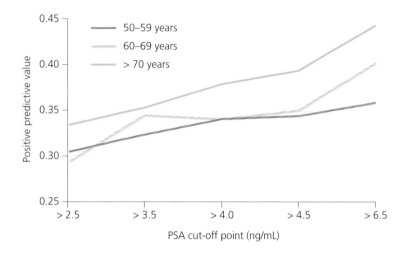

Figure 3.5 Raising the PSA cut-off point in older men increases the positive predictive value, but reduces the overall detection rate.

Screening

The value of screening asymptomatic men for prostate cancer is controversial (Table 3.6). As described in Chapter 1, there is a great discrepancy between the incidence of clinically significant disease and the prevalence of microscopic disease, and identification of those men in whom disease progression is probable remains inexact. Preliminary results from two major randomized trials testing whether prostate cancer screening reduces mortality have recently been reported (see page 32), but neither is fully mature yet. Unfortunately, the results are conflicting and until the full data are available the practice of screening will remain controversial. Current evidence to support screening of men for prostate cancer is as follows.

- Non-randomized data show that since the advent of PSA screening in the USA and Europe, the proportion of men presenting with advanced prostate cancer has decreased, as has prostate cancer mortality.
- Men with localized prostate cancer treated with radical prostatectomy have a 44% reduction in risk of premature death compared with conservative management.

35

TABLE 3.6

Screening for prostate cancer

Pros

- Simple tests available (PSA and DRE)
- Detects early, potentially curable lesions
- Reassures those who are screened as negative
- Screening reduces mortality by 27%

Cons

- False-positive findings cause anxiety
- Biopsy guided by transrectal ultrasonography carries a 2% risk of serious infective complications
- Expensive
- Some small, slow-growing cancers will be treated unnecessarily, and treatment has side effects

- The PSA test and DRE are simple to perform and the prostate biopsy has a low complication rate.

Disadvantages to screening include the following.

- There is a potential to detect and treat clinically insignificant cancers that are better left undetected.
- There is a morbidity associated with prostate cancer treatments.
- A large proportion of men having a biopsy will not harbor prostate cancer.
- The screening process may generate anxiety.

Prostate cancer screening potentially has the greatest benefit in younger men, who have a greater life-expectancy. Groups that advocate screening generally suggest screening between the ages of 40 and 70 years. Screening is generally not beneficial in elderly men or men with significant comorbidities, who have reduced life-expectancy and are likely to die from other causes.

The family physician has an important role in assessing the likely benefits and risks for individual patients according to their age and life-expectancy; appropriate counseling of the patient and his immediate family is an essential element of this process.

Clinical symptoms

Patients with prostate cancer may present with a variety of symptoms (Table 3.7).

Localized cancer. When the cancer is localized, it is generally asymptomatic. Men will often present with symptoms of BPH that are unrelated to the cancer. These symptoms occur when benign prostatic tissue compresses and obstructs the urethra, resulting in frequency, hesitancy and poor flow. Prostate cancer may also present as an 'incidental' finding after TURP (Figure 3.6); nowadays, less than 10% of men undergoing TURP for BPH are found to have microscopic foci of prostate cancer.

TABLE 3.7

Clinical presentation/symptoms of local and locally invasive prostate cancer

Local disease	Locally invasive disease
• Asymptomatic	• Hematuria
• Elevated PSA	• Dysuria
• BPH symptoms	• Perineal and suprapubic pain
– weak stream	• Erectile dysfunction
– hesitancy	• Incontinence
– sensation of incomplete emptying	• Loin pain or anuria resulting from obstruction of the ureters
– frequency	• Symptoms of renal failure
– urgency	• Hemospermia
– urge incontinence	• Rectal symptoms, including tenesmus
– urinary tract infection	

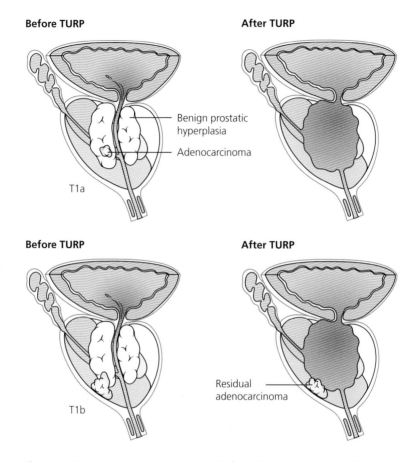

Figure 3.6 Prostate cancer is occasionally found in resected chips of prostate tissue obtained during TURP in up to 10% of cases. About two-thirds of these are well-differentiated T1a lesions involving less than 5% of the chips. The remaining lesions are larger volume, less well differentiated T1b cancers. A number of potential sampling errors are inherent in the diagnosis of prostate cancer at TURP. T1a tumors that are confined to the transition zone may be completely excised, whereas significant amounts of T1b tumors may remain after the procedure.

Locally advanced cancers (usually palpable by DRE) may cause symptoms resulting from local extension of the tumor, such as irritative symptoms (frequency, urgency) that can occur as a result of invasion of the bladder trigone and pelvic nerves. Involvement of the perineal or suprapubic nerves can lead to pain, and thus the possibility of prostate cancer should be considered in the investigation of prostatitis-like symptoms.

Hematuria can occur from erosion of the cancer into the urethra or bladder. Loin pain can occur because of ureteric obstruction and hydronephrosis. Symptoms of bladder outlet obstruction can occur when a large cancer obstructs the bladder outlet, similar to BPH. Invasion of the urethral sphincter or, more commonly, surgery itself may cause urinary incontinence. It is important to exclude the possibility that incontinence is a result of chronic urinary retention with overflow, which may be treatable with procedures such as TURP. Constipation, tenesmus and rectal bleeding can present as a result of the large prostate protruding into the rectal lumen. Invasion of the seminal vesicles may occasionally result in hemospermia, but this is not a common symptom.

Metastatic disease. The most common presenting symptoms are shown in Table 3.8. Pain resulting from bony metastases, particularly in the pelvis and lumbar spine, is the major symptom; thus, the sudden onset of progressive low back or pelvic pain is an important diagnostic feature of metastatic prostate cancer. Pathological fractures may also

TABLE 3.8

Presenting symptoms of metastatic prostate cancer

Distant metastases

- Bone pain or sciatica
- Paraplegia secondary to spinal cord compression
- Lymph node enlargement
- Loin pain or anuria due to obstruction of the ureters by lymph nodes

Widespread metastases

- Lethargy (e.g. due to anemia or uremia)
- Weight loss and cachexia
- Cutaneous and bowel hemorrhage (unusual)

occur, particularly affecting the neck of the femur. Metastases within the vertebrae, sometimes leading to spinal cord compression, are not uncommon and may produce backache or neurological symptoms in up to 12% of affected men.

Metastasis into the lymph nodes may result in lymph node enlargement. Intra-abdominal lymph node metastasis usually begins in the obturator and internal iliac nodes, spreads to the iliac nodes and beyond and may, with local tumors, result in obstruction of the ureters. In advanced disease, lymphatic involvement may extend to the thoracic, cervical, inguinal and axillary nodes. Lymph node metastases may produce a number of symptoms, including palpable swellings, loin pain or anuria due to obstruction of the ureters, and swelling of the lower limbs as a result of lymphedema.

Systemic metastases in the liver, lungs or elsewhere may produce non-specific symptoms, such as lethargy resulting from anemia or uremia, weight loss and cachexia.

Key points – screening and presentation

- Increasingly, prostate cancer is being diagnosed on the basis of raised PSA values.
- PSA-based screening of asymptomatic men is controversial.
- Transrectal ultrasound-guided biopsies are needed to confirm the diagnosis.
- More advanced disease can present with symptoms of bladder outflow obstruction.
- Bone metastases may cause bone pain or pathological fracture.

Key references

Andriole GL, Crawford ED, Grubb RL 3rd et al. Mortality results from a randomized prostate-cancer screening trial. *N Engl J Med* 2009;360: 1310–19.

Benson MC, Whang IS, Olsson CA et al. The use of prostate specific antigen density to enhance the predictive value of intermediate levels of serum prostate specific antigen. *J Urol* 1992;147:817–21.

Berger AP, Deibl M, Strasak A et al. Large-scale study of clinical impact of PSA velocity: long-term PSA kinetics as method of differentiating men with from those without prostate cancer. *Urology* 2007;69: 134–8.

Bratslavsky G, Fisher HA, Kaufman RP Jr, Voskoboynik D, Nazeer T, Mian BM. PSA-related markers in the detection of prostate cancer and high-grade disease in the contemporary era with extended biopsy. *Urol Oncol* 2008;26:166–70.

Brawer MK. Clinical usefulness of assays for complexed prostate-specific antigen. *Urol Clin North Am* 2002;29:193–203.

Catalona WJ, Smith DS, Ornstein DK. Prostate cancer detection in men with serum PSA concentrations of 2.6 to 4.0 ng/mL and benign prostate examination. Enhancement of specificity with free PSA measurements. *JAMA* 1997; 277:1452–5.

Chun FK, Hutterer GC, Perrotte P et al. Distribution of prostate specific antigen (PSA) and percentage free PSA in a contemporary screening cohort with no evidence of prostate cancer. *BJU Int* 2007;100:37–41.

D'Amico AV, Chen MH, Roehl KA et al. Preoperative PSA velocity and the risk of death from prostate cancer after radical prostatectomy. *N Engl J Med* 2004;351:125–35.

D'Amico AV, Renshaw AA, Sussman B et al. Pretreatment PSA velocity and the risk of death from prostate cancer following external beam radiotherapy. *JAMA* 2005;294:440–7.

de Koning HJ, Auvinen A, Berenguer Sanchez A et al. Large-scale randomized prostate cancer screening trials: program performances in the European Randomized Screening for Prostate Cancer trial and the Prostate, Lung, Colorectal and Ovary cancer trial. *Int J Cancer* 2002;97:237–44.

de Koning HJ, Liem MK, Baan CA et al. Prostate cancer mortality reduction by screening: power and time frame with complete enrollment in the European Randomised Screening for Prostate Cancer (ERSPC) trial. *Int J Cancer* 2002;98:268–73.

Gann PH, Ma J, Catalona WJ, Stampfer MJ. Strategies combining total and percent free prostate specific antigen for detecting prostate cancer: a prospective evaluation. *J Urol* 2002;167:2427–34.

Gleason DF, Mellinger GT. Prediction of prognosis for prostatic adenocarcinoma by combined histological grading and clinical staging. 1974. *J Urol* 2002;167: 953–8; discussion 959.

Grubb RL 3rd, Pinsky PF, Greenlee RT et al. Prostate cancer screening in the Prostate, Lung, Colorectal and Ovarian cancer screening trial: update on findings from the initial four rounds of screening in a randomized trial. *BJU Int* 2008; 102:1524–30.

Loeb S, Roehl KA, Antenor JA et al. Prostate-specific antigen compared with median prostate-specific antigen for age group as predictor of prostate cancer risk in men younger than 60 years old. *Urology* 2006;67:316–20.

Loeb S, Roehl KA, Catalona WJ, Nadler RB. Is the utility of prostate-specific antigen velocity for prostate cancer detection affected by age? *BJU Int* 2008;101:817–21.

Nixon RG, Brawer MK. Enhancing the specificity of prostate-specific antigen: an overview of PSA density, PSA velocity and age-specific PSA reference ranges. *Br J Urol* 1997; 79:61–7.

Oesterling JE, Jacobsen SJ, Chute CG et al. Serum prostate-specific antigen in a community-based population of healthy men. Establishment of age-specific reference ranges. *JAMA* 1993;270:860–4.

Okihara K, Cheli CD, Partin AW et al. Comparative analysis of complexed prostate specific antigen, free prostate specific antigen and their ratio in detecting prostate cancer. *J Urol* 2002;167:2017–23.

Parkes C, Wald NJ, Murphy P et al. Prospective observational study to assess value of PSA as screening test for prostate cancer. *BMJ* 1995;311: 1340–3.

Partin AW, Brawer MK, Subong ENP et al. Prospective evaluation of percent free-PSA and complexed-PSA for early detection of prostate cancer. *Prostate Cancer Prostatic Dis* 1998; 1:197–203.

Punglia RS, D'Amico AV, Catalona WJ et al. Effect of verification bias on screening for prostate cancer by measurement of prostate-specific antigen. *N Engl J Med* 2003;349:335–42.

Schröder FH, Hugosson J, Roobol MJ et al. Screening and prostate-cancer mortality in a randomized European study. *N Engl J Med* 2009;360:1320-8.

Schröder FH, Wildhagen MF. Screening for prostate cancer: evidence and perspectives. *BJU Int* 2001;88:811–17.

Thompson IM, Pauler DK, Goodman PJ et al. Prevalence of prostate cancer among men with a prostate-specific antigen level < or = 4.0 ng per milliliter. *N Engl J Med* 2004;350: 2239–46.

Van Cangh PJ, Nayer PD, Sauvage P. Free to total PSA ratio is superior to total PSA in differentiating BPH from prostate cancer. *Prostate* 1996;7:30–4.

Van Der Cruijsen-Koeter IW, Wildhagen MF, De Koning HJ, Schroder FH. The value of current diagnostic tests in prostate cancer screening. *BJU Int* 2001;88:458–66.

Woodrum DL, Brawer MK, Partin AW et al. Interpretation of free prostate-specific antigen clinical research studies for the detection of prostate cancer. *J Urol* 1998;159: 5–12.

Prognostic indicators and staging

Accurate grading and staging of prostate cancer, particularly distinguishing between Gleason grades and between localized and extensive disease, is important for selection of the best treatment option. Although developments in imaging techniques have led to more accurate staging than can be achieved with digital rectal examination (DRE) or prostate-specific antigen (PSA) testing alone, both under- and overstaging are still common clinical problems. Thus, a need remains not only for improved staging techniques, but also for better prognostic indicators.

Staging of localized disease

Staging of localized disease relies primarily on the following techniques:
- DRE
- PSA measurement
- transrectal ultrasonography (TRUS) and ultrasound-guided biopsy
- computerized tomography (CT) scanning
- magnetic resonance imaging (MRI)
- tables and nomograms to predict disease stage and outcome.

Digital rectal examination. The accuracy of DRE in staging prostate cancer is 30–50%; underestimation is common because small and anteriorly located tumors are generally impalpable, and false-positive findings may occur in patients with conditions such as BPH or prostatitis. The technique can, however, detect a number of significant cancers when PSA is still within the normal range (< 4.0 ng/mL) and provide useful, if imprecise, information about the local stage of the disease (Table 4.1).

Prostate-specific antigen determination. Within groups of patients, there is a reasonable correlation between PSA levels and the pathological stage (and, to a lesser extent, the clinical stage) of prostate cancer. The correlation is poorer, however, in individual patients because of the

TABLE 4.1

Clinical local staging of prostate cancer by DRE

Tumor stage	DRE findings
T2a	Peripheral, firm nodule; no apparent distortion of capsule
T2b	Hard, more irregular; unilateral enlargement may be present
T3	Irregular distortion; prostate remains mobile; seminal vesicles may be palpable
T4	Gross enlargement; hard and irregular; prostate immobile owing to invasion to surrounding tissues

considerable overlap between the PSA ranges associated with different stages. PSA levels above 20 ng/mL are often indicative of tumor extension beyond the prostatic capsule, while levels above 40 ng/mL suggest a high likelihood of bony or soft tissue metastases (Tables 4.2 and 4.3, and Figure 4.1).

PSA velocity has also been shown to be helpful in identifying men with aggressive disease. A recent study observed that men who had a velocity above 2.0 ng/mL/year immediately before diagnosis were at high risk of death from prostate cancer, irrespective of treatment.

Although the serum PSA concentration alone may not be a precise indicator of stage on an individual basis, it can sometimes be used to eliminate some staging investigations. It appears that men who present with newly diagnosed, well- or moderately well-differentiated prostate cancer, no skeletal symptoms and a serum PSA value less than or equal to 10 ng/mL may not always need a staging radionuclide bone scan. For these individuals, the probability of having skeletal metastases approaches zero. Many clinicians, however, still like to use this test as a baseline investigation because it may identify 'hot spots' due to conditions such as degenerative osteoarthritis that may cause confusion later – if or when the PSA level starts to rise. A negative scan also serves to reassure a patient that his skeleton is not involved.

TABLE 4.2

Partin's table* relating PSA, tumor grade and clinical stage to the probability (%) of extraprostatic extension, seminal vesicle involvement or lymph node involvement for men with clinically normal rectal examination

PSA range (ng/mL)	Pathological stage	Gleason score				
		2–4	5–6	3 + 4 = 7	4 + 3 = 7	8–10
0–2.5	Organ confined	95 (89–99)	90 (88–93)	79 (74–85)	71 (62–79)	66 (54–76)
	Extraprostatic extension	5 (1–11)	9 (7–12)	17 (13–23)	25 (18–34)	28 (20–38)
	Seminal vesicle (+)	–	0 (0–1)	2 (1–5)	2 (1–5)	4 (1–10)
	Lymph node (+)	–	–	1 (0–2)	1 (0–4)	1 (0–4)
2.6–4.0	Organ confined	92 (82–98)	84 (81–86)	68 (62–74)	58 (48–67)	52 (41–63)
	Extraprostatic extension	8 (2–18)	15 (13–18)	27 (22–33)	37 (29–46)	40 (31–50)
	Seminal vesicle (+)	–	1 (0–1)	4 (2–7)	4 (1–7)	6 (3–12)
	Lymph node (+)	–	–	1 (0–2)	1 (0–3)	1 (0–4)
4.1–6.0	Organ confined	90 (78–98)	80 (78–83)	63 (58–68)	52 (43–60)	46 (36–56)
	Extraprostatic extension	10 (2–22)	19 (16–21)	32 (27–36)	42 (35–50)	45 (36–54)
	Seminal vesicle (+)	–	1 (0–1)	3 (2–5)	3 (1–6)	5 (3–9)
	Lymph node (+)	–	0 (0–1)	2 (1–3)	3 (1–5)	3 (1–6)
6.1–10.0	Organ confined	87 (73–97)	75 (72–77)	54 (49–59)	43 (35–51)	37 (28–46)
	Extraprostatic extension	13 (3–27)	23 (21–25)	36 (32–40)	47 (40–54)	48 (39–57)
	Seminal vesicle (+)	–	2 (2–3)	8 (6–11)	8 (4–12)	13 (8–19)
	Lymph node (+)	–	0 (0–1)	2 (1–3)	2 (1–4)	3 (1–5)
> 10.0	Organ confined	80 (61–95)	62 (58–64)	37 (32–42)	27 (21–34)	22 (16–30)
	Extraprostatic extension	20 (5–39)	33 (30–36)	43 (38–48)	51 (44–59)	50 (42–59)
	Seminal vesicle (+)	–	4 (3–5)	12 (9–17)	11 (6–17)	17 (10–25)
	Lymph node (+)	–	2 (1–3)	8 (5–11)	10 (5–17)	11 (5–18)

*Partin's tables are based on the retrospective analysis of several thousand patients undergoing radical prostatectomy.

TABLE 4.3

Partin's table* relating PSA, tumor grade and clinical stage to the probability (%) of extraprostatic extension, seminal vesicle involvement or lymph node involvement for men with clinically palpable tumours (cT2a)

PSA range (ng/mL)	Pathological stage	Gleason score				
		2–4	5–6	3 + 4 = 7	4 + 3 = 7	8–10
0–2.5	Organ confined	86 (71–97)	73 (63–81)	51 (38–63)	39 (26–54)	34 (21–48)
	Extraprostatic extension	14 (3–29)	24 (17–33)	36 (26–48)	45 (32–59)	47 (33–61)
	Seminal vesicle (+)	–	1 (0–4)	5 (1–13)	5 (1–12)	8 (2–19)
	Lymph node (+)	–	1 (0–4)	6 (0–18)	9 (0–26)	10 (0–27)
2.6–4.0	Organ confined	78 (58–94)	61 (50–70)	38 (27–50)	27 (18–40)	23 (14–34)
	Extraprostatic extension	22 (6–42)	36 (27–45)	48 (37–59)	57 (44–70)	57 (44–70)
	Seminal vesicle (+)	–	2 (1–5)	8 (2–17)	6 (2–16)	10 (3–22)
	Lymph node (+)	–	1 (0–4)	5 (0–15)	7 (0–21)	8 (0–22)
4.1–6.0	Organ confined	73 (52–93)	55 (44–64)	31 (23–41)	21 (14–31)	18 (11–28)
	Extraprostatic extension	27 (7–48)	40 (32–50)	50 (40–60)	57 (43–68)	57 (43–70)
	Seminal vesicle (+)	–	2 (1–4)	6 (2–11)	4 (1–10)	7 (2–15)
	Lymph node (+)	–	3 (1–7)	12 (5–23)	16 (6–32)	16 (6–33)
6.1–10.0	Organ confined	67 (45–91)	46 (36–56)	24 (17–32)	16 (10–24)	13 (8–20)
	Extraprostatic extension	33 (9–55)	46 (37–55)	52 (42–61)	58 (46–69)	56 (43–69)
	Seminal vesicle (+)	–	5 (2–9)	13 (6–23)	11 (4–21)	16 (6–29)
	Lymph node (+)	–	3 (1–6)	10 (5–18)	13 (6–25)	13 (5–26)
> 10.0	Organ confined	54 (32–85)	30 (21–38)	11 (7–17)	7 (4–12)	6 (3–10)
	Extraprostatic extension	46 (15–68)	51 (42–60)	42 (30–55)	43 (29–59)	41 (27–57)
	Seminal vesicle (+)	–	6 (2–12)	13 (6–24)	10 (3–20)	15 (5–28)
	Lymph node (+)	–	13 (6–22)	33 (18–49)	38 (20–58)	38 (20–59)

*Partin's tables are based on the retrospective analysis of several thousand patients undergoing radical prostatectomy.

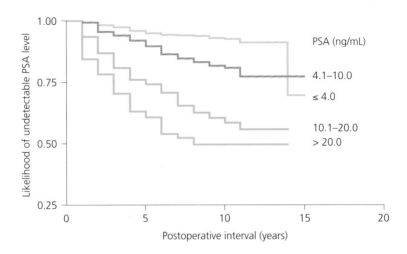

Figure 4.1 Kaplan–Meier actuarial likelihood of PSA-free progression after radical prostatectomy by preoperative serum PSA levels.

Transrectal ultrasonography has a number of uses in the management of prostate cancer. It is most commonly used to image the prostate gland and direct the biopsy sampling device to the appropriate spot during prostate biopsy (Figure 4.2). Antibiotics are given before and after the procedure to reduce the risk of infection, currently estimated at around 2%. A quinolone is the usual choice, though quinolone resistance appears to be increasing. Usually 8–14 TRUS-guided biopsies are taken from different regions of the prostate with an 18-gauge needle. This is now routinely performed on an outpatient basis, preferably after infiltration with local anesthesia. The percentage of each biopsy core involved and the overall number of positive biopsy specimens provide a useful estimate of tumor volume (Figure 4.3). In high-risk cases (large, bulky, palpable tumors, or PSA > 20 ng/mL), additional lateral capsular and seminal vesicle biopsies can be taken with minimal extra morbidity to confirm or exclude extraprostatic extension.

TRUS is also used to measure the volume of the prostate gland prior to biopsy. This can be useful for calculating the PSA density.

Cancer within the prostate gland is not usually apparent ultrasonographically, but occasionally can present with a number of ultrasonographic abnormalities. These include abnormal echo patterns

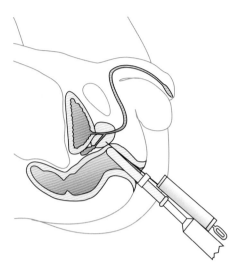

Figure 4.2 TRUS-guided biopsy. An ultrasound probe is introduced into the rectum to lie adjacent to the prostate. Under antibiotic cover and ultrasound control, multiple prostatic biopsies may be taken with an automatic biopsy gun.

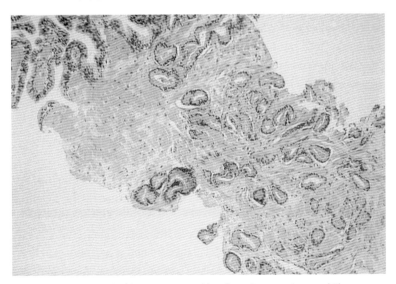

Figure 4.3 A prostatic biopsy core positive for adenocarcinoma (Gleason grades 3 and 4, Gleason score 7).

49

(usually hypoechoic); loss of differentiation between central and peripheral zones; asymmetry of size or shape; and capsular distortion.

Some prostate tumours are hypoechoic but hypoechoic images may result from other causes, so the specificity of this finding for prostate cancer is only 20–25%. Assessment of local staging by TRUS imaging alone is poor. When extracapsular extension or seminal vesicle extension is suspected on imaging, a biopsy of the area is required for confirmation.

CT scanning has virtually no role in the local staging of prostate cancer, as separation from surrounding muscle is poor and intraprostatic anatomy is not well defined. Its primary role is in the detection of nodal metastases. The sensitivity of this modality is reported typically at 36%, because the criterion for detection of positive disease is based on nodal size (> 10 mm) and CT is not able to detect microscopic nodal metastases, which are much more common. Although CT can be used to monitor bone metastases, bone scans and MRI are far superior.

Magnetic resonance imaging with an endorectal coil has been used to detect prostate cancer, but it is not widely utilized because its accuracy is debated. MRI for the staging of prostate cancer is also controversial. On MRI, criteria for extracapsular extension include asymmetry, irregular speculated prostate margin and obliterated recto-prostatic angle. The sensitivity of MRI for the detection of extracapsular extension has been reported to range from 13% to 95%, and accuracy is certainly higher in large units with a lot of experience in interpreting prostate images. MRI has no advantage over CT in the evaluation of nodal metastases. However, promising results have been reported with the use of ultrasmall superparamagnetic iron oxide particles as an aid to nodal metastasis evaluation by MRI.

The addition of magnetic resonance (MR) spectroscopy (evaluation of chemical metabolites in a small volume of interest by MR technology) has also improved the accuracy of MR staging. Dynamic contrast-enhanced MRI is a method of imaging the prostate during rapid infusion of gadolinium contrast. Prostate cancer is detected based on early enhancement resulting from angiogenesis. While this enhancement is typical, it is not specific and has a sensitivity of 73% in defining prostate cancer.

Prognostic tables and nomograms. While cancer characteristics such as PSA, Gleason score, clinical stage, number of biopsy cores involved and percentage of each core involved provide valuable prognostic information, combining all of these variables in a nomogram gives a much more accurate prediction of the patient's outcome. Many of these nomograms are available on the web or for use on personal digital assistants (PDAs). Nomograms have been developed, based on the data from thousands of patients, that predict the pathological likelihood of seminal vesicle invasion, lymph node metastasis and extracapsular extension on each side or presence of a small, insignificant cancer. Other nomograms have been developed to predict the likelihood of recurrence of cancer after treatment by radical prostatectomy, external-beam radiotherapy and brachytherapy. More simple prediction tools, such as Partin's tables (Tables 4.2 and 4.3), tabulate the likely pathology from categorical values of PSA, Gleason score and clinical stage. These readily available clinical predictors are very useful for patient counseling and making treatment decisions, as well as for planning treatment such as surgery.

Staging of metastatic disease

Staging of metastatic disease involves assessing the extent of bone and soft tissue involvement. The principal techniques used are a chest X-ray, radionuclide bone scanning, CT and MRI.

Radionuclide bone scanning is usually performed as a baseline assessment at the time of the initial diagnosis of prostate cancer (Figure 4.4). If the PSA value is less than 10 ng/mL and the Gleason score is below 8, it may be permissible to omit this test as it is rarely positive in these circumstances. The use of this technique in routine follow-up has declined as PSA measurements have been shown to be the most accurate and cost-effective means of monitoring bony metastases.

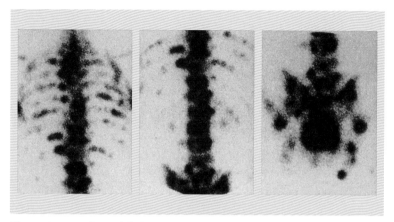

Figure 4.4 A radionuclide bone scan showing multiple bony metastases resulting from disseminated prostate cancer.

CT scanning of the abdomen and pelvis may be used in cases in which treatment decisions depend on the presence and degree of lymph node involvement. Small-volume and microscopic metastases (< 1 cm) are not usually detectable by this technique, and thus the accuracy of CT scanning is only 40–50%. CT scanning may also be employed occasionally to guide fine needle aspiration of enlarged lymph nodes for cytological analysis to aid diagnosis.

Magnetic resonance imaging can also be used to identify metastatic disease affecting the regional lymph nodes. However, most scanners do not permit guided fine needle aspiration, and MRI is often omitted if the PSA is below 10 ng/mL. MRI may also be useful for clarifying the nature of any abnormality in equivocal bone scans and, importantly, for recognizing incipient spinal cord compression.

Immunoscintigraphy using radioactive antibodies directed against prostate-specific proteins has proved inadequate for clinical use in its present form owing to its lack of specificity and sensitivity.

Approach to staging

An approach to the diagnosis and staging of localized prostate cancer is outlined in Figure 4.5.

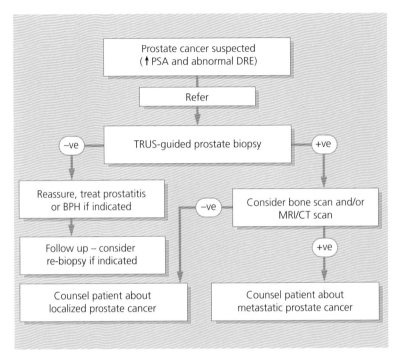

Figure 4.5 Algorithm for diagnosis and staging of prostate cancer.

Key points – prognostic indicators and staging

- Prostate cancer is usually diagnosed on the basis of TRUS-guided biopsies under antibiotic cover and local anesthesia.
- The Gleason score of these biopsies, the clinical stage on DRE and the presenting PSA value provide an estimate of the risk of extraprostatic extension.
- MRI can provide information about local staging.
- Bone scanning identifies bone metastases, but the probability of these with PSA < 10 ng/mL is low.

Key references

Alonzi R, Padhani AR, Allen C. Dynamic contrast enhanced MRI in prostate cancer. *Eur J Radiol* 2007;63:335–50.

Cagiannos I, Karakiewicz P, Eastham JA et al. A preoperative nomogram identifying decreased risk of positive pelvic lymph nodes in patients with prostate cancer. *J Urol* 2003;170: 1798–803.

D'Amico AV, Chen MH, Roehl KA, Catalona WJ. Preoperative PSA velocity and the risk of death from prostate cancer after radical prostatectomy. *N Engl J Med* 2004;351:125–35.

Davis M, Sofer M, Kim SS, Soloway MS. The procedure of transrectal ultrasound guided biopsy of the prostate: a survey of patient preparation and biopsy technique. *J Urol* 2002;167:566–70.

Gleason DF. Histologic grading in clinical staging of prostatic carcinoma. In: Tannenbaum M, ed. *Urologic Pathology: The Prostate.* Philadelphia: Lea & Febiger, 1977:171–98.

Harisinghani MG, Barentsz J, Hahn PF et al. Noninvasive detection of clinically occult lymph-node metastases in prostate cancer. *N Engl J Med* 2003;348:2491–9.

Hricak H, Choyke PL, Eberhardt SC et al. Imaging prostate cancer: a multidisciplinary perspective. *Radiology* 2007;243:28–53.

Ishizuka O, Tanabe T, Nakayama T, Kawakami M, Kinebuchi Y, Nishizawa O. Prostate-specific antigen, Gleason sum and clinical T stage for predicting the need for radionuclide bone scan for prostate cancer patients in Japan. *Int J Urol* 2005;12:728–32.

Kattan MW, Eastham JA, Wheeler TM et al. Counseling men with prostate cancer: a nomogram for predicting the presence of small, moderately differentiated, confined tumors. *J Urol* 2003; 170:1792–7.

Kattan MW, Zelefsky MJ, Kupelian PA et al. Pretreatment nomogram that predicts 5-year probability of metastasis following three-dimensional conformal radiation therapy for localized prostate cancer. *J Clin Oncol* 2003;21:4568–71.

Makarov DV, Sanderson H, Partin AW, Epstein JI. Gleason score 7 prostate cancer on needle biopsy: is the prognostic difference in Gleason scores 4 + 3 and 3 + 4 independent of the number of involved cores? *J Urol* 2002;167:2440–2.

Moul JW, Kane CJ, Malkowicz SB. The role of imaging studies and molecular markers for selecting candidates for radical prostatectomy. *Urol Clin North Am* 2001;28:459–72.

Narain V, Bianco FJ Jr, Grignon DJ et al. How accurately does prostate biopsy Gleason score predict pathologic findings and disease free survival? *Prostate* 2001;49:185–90.

Ohori M, Kattan MW, Koh H et al. Predicting the presence and side of extracapsular extension: a nomogram for staging prostate cancer. *J Urol* 2004;171:1844–9; discussion 1849.

Partin AW, Mangold LA, Lamm DM et al. Contemporary update of prostate cancer staging nomograms (Partin Tables) for the new millennium. *Urology* 2001;58:843–8.

Partin AW, Natlan MW, Subong ENP. Combination of prostate specific antigen, clinical stage and Gleason score to predict pathological stage of localized prostate cancer. *JAMA* 1997;277: 1445–51.

Stephenson AJ, Kattan MW. Nomograms for prostate cancer. *BJU Int* 2006;98:39–46.

Taneja SS, Hsu EI, Cheli CD et al. Complexed prostate-specific antigen as a staging tool: results based on a multicenter prospective evaluation of complexed prostate-specific antigen in cancer diagnosis. *Urology* 2002;60(suppl 1):10–17.

Wang L, Hricak H, Kattan MW et al. Prediction of organ-confined prostate cancer: incremental value of MR imaging and MR spectroscopic imaging to staging nomograms. *Radiology* 2006; 238:597–603

Wolf JS Jr, Cher M, Dall'era M et al. The use and accuracy of cross-sectional imaging and fine needle aspiration cytology for detection of pelvic lymph node metastases before radical prostatectomy. *J Urol* 1995;153:993–9.

Management of localized prostate cancer

The aim of treatment in patients with localized prostate cancer is usually cure – whether eliminating the tumor or preventing death from prostate cancer (as opposed to death with prostate cancer). Figure 5.1 shows the likelihood of a man with localized prostate cancer dying from prostate cancer compared with dying from other causes, stratified by Gleason score and patient's age. Other confounding variables that affect the likelihood of death from prostate cancer include comorbidities, clinical stage and PSA level.

As men with localized disease often do not experience significant disease-related morbidity for several years after diagnosis, and curative treatment itself may result in some morbidity, those with a shorter life-expectancy are likely to benefit least from radical treatment. Table 5.1 lists the treatment options available for localized prostate cancer in men at low-, intermediate- and high-risk of recurrence. These risk groups are based on Gleason score, PSA level and clinical stage. Unfortunately, our knowledge is such that it is not always possible to say which of the treatments will produce the optimum outcome for an individual patient.

Radical prostatectomy involves surgically removing the entire prostate, the seminal vesicles and a variable amount of adjacent tissue (Figure 5.2). It is appropriate for men for whom it is believed the tumor can be removed completely by surgery, and who satisfy the criteria in Table 5.2. The procedure is most commonly performed via the retropubic route – increasingly using laparoscopic technology with or without robotic assistance – though the perineal approach can also be used. The major advantage of radical prostatectomy is that it excises all prostatic tissue and provides precise histological information and definitive cure in patients in whom the tumor is specimen-confined. Thus, the patient's anxiety is relieved during the postoperative period; given that prostate cancer has a long natural history, this is an

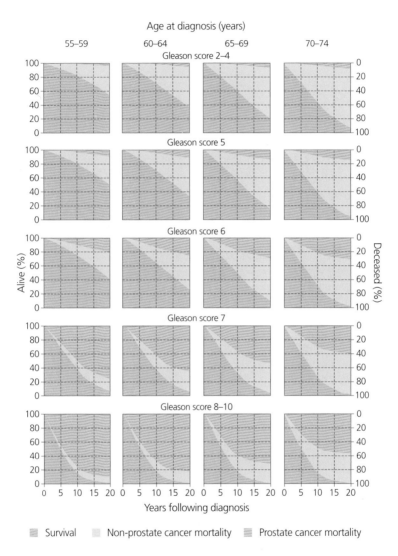

Figure 5.1 Survival and cumulative mortality from prostate cancer and other causes for up to 20 years after diagnosis of localized prostate cancer. Reproduced with permission from Albertsen et al. 2005.

important consideration in terms of the patient's quality of life. Long-term studies have shown normal life-expectancies in those with complete excision of specimen-confined disease. Ten-year survival for

57

TABLE 5.1

Treatment options for localized and locally advanced prostate cancer

Treatment	Localized Risk of recurrence			Locally advanced
	Low	Intermediate	High	
Radical prostatectomy	✓	✓	✓	Multimodality therapy
External-beam radiotherapy	✓	✓		
External-beam radiotherapy with androgen deprivation		✓	✓	✓
Low-dose seed brachytherapy	✓			
Active surveillance	✓			
Watchful waiting	✓	✓	✓	✓
HDR brachytherapy (in combination with external-beam radiotherapy)			✓	✓
Hormonal therapy			✓	✓

Approaches under investigation

HIFU	✓			
Cryotherapy	✓			

HDR, high-dose-rate; HIFU, high-intensity focused ultrasound.

men with clinically localized disease treated with radical prostatectomy is 98%, 91% and 76% for Gleason scores 2–4, 5–7 and 8–10, respectively. Moreover, the procedure also offers definitive treatment of concomitant BPH.

The principal adverse events associated with radical prostatectomy are persistent urinary incontinence (< 2–3%) and erectile dysfunction (> 50%); the latter is age-related, tends to improve with time and can be

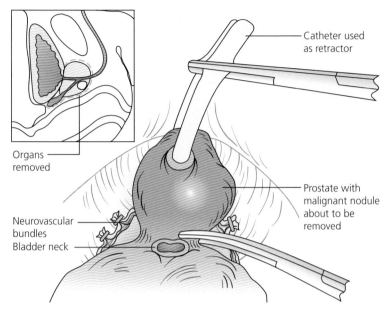

Catheter used
as retractor

Organs
removed

Prostate with
malignant nodule
about to be
removed

Neurovascular
bundles

Bladder neck

Figure 5.2 Radical prostatectomy. The entire prostate and attached seminal vesicles can be removed surgically and an anastomosis created between the bladder neck and the urethra.

TABLE 5.2

Selection criteria for radical prostatectomy

- Histological evidence of prostate cancer
- Clinically localized disease (stages T1–T2)
- Life expectancy > 10 years
- No contraindications to surgery
- No significant comorbidity

---

minimized by nerve-sparing approaches. Moreover, erectile dysfunction after surgery can now be treated effectively (see Chapter 9). Table 5.3 summarizes the advantages and disadvantages of radical prostatectomy.

Radical prostatectomy, by whichever means achieved, is believed by many urologists to offer the best opportunity for cure in patients with

TABLE 5.3

Advantages and disadvantages of radical prostatectomy, radiotherapy and brachytherapy in the treatment of localized prostate cancer

Radical prostatectomy

Advantages

- High likelihood of cure if tumor pathologically confined
- Definitive staging possible
- Treatment of concomitant BPH
- Reliable PSA suppression to unrecordable levels
- Side effects improve with time
- Easy monitoring for recurrent disease
- Radiotherapy possible after surgery

Disadvantages

- Major operation
- Potential mortality (< 0.4%)
- Potential morbidity:
  - impotence (> 50%)
  - persistent incontinence (< 3%)
  - pulmonary embolism (< 1%)
  - bladder neck stricture (< 5%)

Radiotherapy

Advantages

- Potential cure
- Surgery avoided
- Outpatient therapy

Disadvantages

- Prostate left in situ
- Difficulty assessing cure
- No definitive staging possible
- No benefit for concomitant BPH
- Patient anxiety during follow-up

- Unreliable PSA suppression
- May need androgen deprivation in combination
- Potential morbidity:
  - rectal injury (2–10%)
  - urinary incontinence (< 3%)
  - impotence (20–30%)
  - bladder damage (10–20%)
  - hematuria (5–10%)
- Surgery not feasible after radiotherapy

(CONTINUED)

TABLE 5.3 (CONTINUED)

Brachytherapy

Advantages	*Disadvantages*
• One-off treatment	• Only appropriate for low-risk disease
• Day-case or overnight procedure	• Cannot be used after previous prostate surgery
• Limited period of catheterization	• Limited experience of long-term effects
• Low risk of incontinence	• Difficulty assessing cure
• Lower risk of erectile dysfunction	• Makes subsequent surgery dangerous
	• Very significant urinary symptoms in first 6 months

localized prostate cancer. A randomized study from Sweden showed that at a median 8.2 years' follow-up, radical prostatectomy decreased prostate-cancer-related mortality by 44% and overall death by 26% when compared with watchful waiting. The difference was largest in men under 65 years of age. Because the total number of prostate-cancer-related deaths was low, it would require 20 men to undergo prostatectomy to save one man from death.

A similar US study, the PIVOT trial, is fully recruited and results will be available in 2009. Meanwhile, it seems reasonable to discuss the option of radical prostatectomy with younger men with clinically localized disease and no significant comorbidity.

Laparoscopic radical prostatectomy is increasingly employed. It can be facilitated by robotic assistance (Figure 5.3). The results of the procedure appear roughly equivalent to those of open radical prostatectomy. The operating time is usually somewhat longer, but blood loss and length of hospital stay are significantly reduced. It remains to be seen whether the greater magnification and more precise instrumentation result in a lower risk of erectile dysfunction but early results are encouraging.

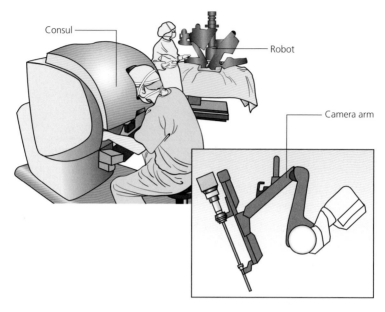

Consul

Robot

Camera arm

Figure 5.3 The *da Vinci* surgical system (Intuitive Surgical, Sunnyvale, California, USA) can be used in laparoscopic radical prostatectomy.

External-beam radiotherapy is widely used in the treatment of localized prostate cancer; it offers a particular advantage in patients who are unsuitable for surgery because of comorbidity or evidence of extraprostatic extension of the cancer. Criteria for patients suitable for radiotherapy are shown in Table 5.4. The treatment generally involves a 7-week course of conformal radiotherapy. Ten-year survival rates of patients undergoing external-beam radiation for clinically localized, prostate cancer with Gleason score 2–4, 5–7 and 8–10 are reported to be approximately 89%, 74% and 52%, respectively.

The principal side effects are due to damage to the bladder, urethra and rectum from radiation scatter. Urinary frequency and urgency are common. Urinary bleeding and pain may occur in severe form in 2–3% of patients. Rectal side effects consist of urgency, frequency and tenesmus. If severe, rectal bleeding, pain or fistula may very occasionally require a colostomy. Erectile dysfunction due to damage to the neurovascular supply to the corpora cavernosa can also occur, often gradually over a 6–18-month period.

TABLE 5.4

Selection criteria for external-beam radiotherapy

- Histological evidence of prostate cancer
- Regionally localized disease
- Sufficient life-expectancy to make cure potentially beneficial
- Absence of lower urinary tract disorders (particularly outflow obstruction)
- Absence of colorectal disease

A number of studies have shown better cancer control for men with intermediate or high-risk prostate cancer if the radiation dose is escalated to 78 Gy or higher. The advent of intensity-modulated radiotherapy (IMRT) allows very precise targeting of the prostate, with less radiation scatter to surrounding organs. As a consequence, higher doses can be given to men without a significant increase in local toxicity. The advantages and disadvantages of radiotherapy are summarized in Table 5.3 and are compared with those of radical prostatectomy and brachytherapy.

Low-dose seed brachytherapy involves placing either iodine-125 or palladium-103 seeds into the prostate via the transperineal route, using a template and TRUS guidance (Figure 5.4). Patient selection criteria are given in Table 5.5. The results of seed brachytherapy in low-risk men (PSA < 10 ng/mL, Gleason score < 7 and ≤ cT2b) is equivalent to radical prostatectomy at 10 years, but they are highly dependent on the quality of seed placement. The results in patients with intermediate risk are worse, however, with freedom from recurrence approximately 66% at 10 years.

The method is gaining popularity, particularly in the USA, because of its low morbidity; the side effects are similar in nature to those of external-beam radiotherapy, but may also include difficulty with urination because of prostate swelling. In general, brachytherapy is not suitable for prostates with volumes greater than 60 cm^3 or in men with severe, pre-existing bladder outflow obstruction.

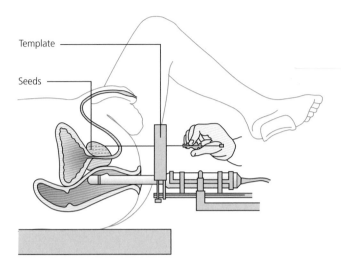

Template

Seeds

Figure 5.4 Brachytherapy.

TABLE 5.5

Selection criteria for low-dose seed brachytherapy

- Histological evidence of prostate cancer
- Clinically localized disease (T1 or T2)
- Low PSA (preferably < 10 ng/mL)
- Low–moderate Gleason score (2–6) preferable
- Prostate volume not large (< 50 cm³)
- Minimal obstructive urinary symptoms
- No prior TURP

Quality-of-life studies performed on men who have undergone surgery, external-beam radiotherapy or seed brachytherapy show no differences in global quality of life between the different modalities.

Active surveillance is reserved for men with small-volume and low-to-moderate-grade prostate cancer, who have a low risk of death from prostate cancer. These men would be eligible for curative therapy based on the criteria discussed earlier, but this option is deferred until objective signs of biological activity are observed. This approach means the majority of men are spared the side effects of curative therapy when they do not require it.

During active surveillance, men are followed closely with regular PSA measurements and DREs on a 3–6-monthly basis. MRI and repeated prostate biopsies are usually organized at 6–12 months following diagnosis and when cancer growth is suspected. Curative therapy is initiated before the cancer becomes incurable. The cancer-specific survival in men who fit the criteria for active surveillance is 99% at 8 years' follow up. While men avoid the physical side effects of cancer treatment, they have to live with the psychological effects of having an untreated cancer.

Watchful waiting is different from active surveillance in that it is for men who are older or who have shorter life-expectancy, and have prostate cancer that is unlikely to shorten their life. These men are counseled and reviewed regularly with clinical examination and PSA measurements. When disease progression is identified, instead of having curative therapy, palliative androgen deprivation is initiated. This is continued until death. In a recent meta-analysis, the development of metastatic disease during watchful waiting was reported to be 2.1% per year in patients with well-differentiated tumors (Gleason scores 2–4), compared with 13.5% per year in patients with aggressive tumors (Gleason scores 7–10). In another study, patients with low-grade tumors treated with watchful waiting had a 92% disease-specific survival at 10 years compared with 76% and 43% for moderate-grade and high-grade tumors, respectively.

High-intensity focused ultrasound (HIFU) technology has been developed to treat localized prostate cancer. A probe delivers HIFU transrectally to the prostate and achieves focal tissue destruction (Figure 5.5). Early results are promising, with 94% of men with low-risk disease reported to be disease free at 3 years' follow up. HIFU can also be used for the treatment of cancer recurrence after radiotherapy. The method should currently be regarded as experimental, particularly

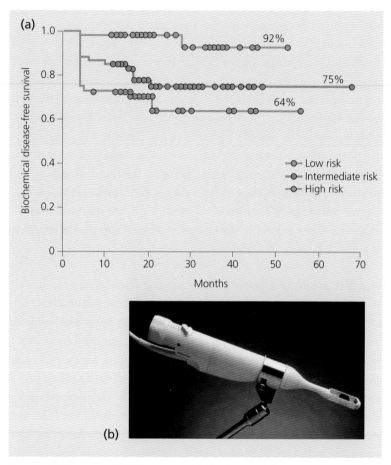

Figure 5.5 Transrectal HIFU therapy: (a) biochemical disease-free survival rate after HIFU therapy, reproduced with permission from Uchida et al. 2006. Copyright Blackwell Publishing; (b) HIFU probe for endorectal treatment of localized prostate cancer.

as side effects of incontinence and the development of urinary fistula may be troublesome and difficult to resolve.

Cryoablation. Freezing temperatures can be used to destroy prostatic tissue. Under TRUS guidance, a number of cryogenic probes are inserted into the prostate via the perineum (Figure 5.6). Liquid nitrogen is then circulated through the probes, producing 'ice balls' with a

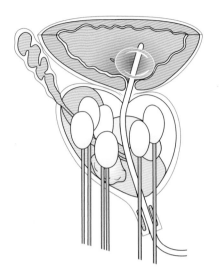

Figure 5.6 In cryoablation, cryogenic probes are inserted into the prostate under ultrasound control, and liquid nitrogen is circulated to destroy prostatic tissue. The urethra is protected by warming through a catheter.

temperature of approximately −180°C that disrupt cell membranes, thereby destroying the surrounding tissue. The urethra is protected by circulating warm (44°C) water through a catheter. Although some studies have reported outcomes comparable to those achieved by radical prostatectomy, others have reported a significant incidence of complications such as rectal and urethral damage. No long-term, randomized, controlled trials have yet compared cryoablation with more established treatments, and the treatment may be more applicable to patients with recurrence after radiotherapy.

Management of high-risk prostate cancer

The term 'high risk' refers to men with prostate cancer who have the cancer still confined to the prostate gland but have a high Gleason score (> 7) or high PSA level (> 20 ng/mL) or men with stage T3/T4N0M0 disease, in which the tumor is no longer confined to the prostate but there is no clinical evidence of spread to local lymph nodes or more distant sites. Both groups of men are at high risk of recurrence following curative therapy. Table 5.6 lists the indicators of poor prognosis that put men at high risk of recurrence.

The treatment options available for men with high-risk prostate cancer are listed in Table 5.1.

67

TABLE 5.6

Poor prognostic factors in prostate cancer

- Gleason sum $\geq$ 8
- Positive seminal vesicle (T3c)
- Invasion of adjacent structures (T4)
- Nodal metastases (N1)
- High PSA (> 20 ng/mL)

The objective of treating men with high-risk prostate cancer is to obtain local control and, ideally, cure.

Watchful waiting. Many patients with high-risk disease are elderly, and thus have a relatively short life-expectancy. Watchful waiting may be a valid treatment option in these patients, who will not infrequently succumb to other comorbid conditions. Patients and their immediate family should be fully informed about the implications of opting for watchful waiting; PSA values should be monitored carefully and symptomatic treatment offered as appropriate.

Hormonal treatment followed by surgery. Hormonal therapy (cytoreduction) for prostate cancer can normally be achieved with luteinizing hormone-releasing hormone (LHRH) analogs together with an antiandrogen to prevent initial androgen stimulation of the tumor ('tumor flare'), thereby reducing the tumor burden. This is sometimes referred to as 'hormonal downstaging'. Such treatment has been shown to reduce PSA levels, prostate volume and tumor volume. Some studies have demonstrated pathological downstaging after endocrine treatment, but this may be partly attributable to poor initial staging of the tumor or difficulties with pathological interpretation. At present, therefore, androgen ablation therapy given neoadjuvantly prior to radical prostatectomy remains an investigational approach pursued by few clinicians. So far, no survival advantage has been reported for this approach, though the incidence of positive surgical margins does appear to be reduced.

Following surgery, patients who have adverse pathological features such as extracapsular extension, seminal vesicle extension or positive margins can be treated with adjuvant radiotherapy to the prostatic bed. In three randomized trials, this has been shown to decrease the risk of PSA recurrence by 52% compared with no treatment. Whether early salvage radiation is equivalent to adjuvant radiation is yet to be answered, and salvage radiotherapy remains an option in these patients (see Chapter 6).

Radiotherapy with hormone therapy. External-beam radiation alone is often inadequate to suppress PSA to within the normal range and prevent disease progression in patients with high-risk disease. Reduction of the tumor burden with an LHRH analog and an antiandrogen may increase the likelihood of totally destroying the remaining cancer cells by irradiation. Hormone therapy also appears to increase the sensitivity of cancer cells to death by irradiation. This approach has been validated in randomized trials, where survival has been shown to improve when men with high-risk prostate cancers are treated with a combination of external-beam radiotherapy and adjuvant hormonal therapy. The addition of adjuvant hormonal therapy improved survival at 5 years from 62% to 78% (Figure 5.7). Similar improvements have been noted in another North American trial, in which prostate cancer mortality was reduced from 31% to 23%. It is now standard practice to add hormonal therapy to the treatment of all men undergoing external-beam radiotherapy for high-risk disease.

High-dose-rate brachytherapy is a new treatment in which a high-intensity iridium source is delivered to the prostate by hollow needles inserted through the perineum (Figure 5.8). It has a number of advantages over low-dose seed brachytherapy.
- The treatment time is very short.
- Very high doses can be achieved in the prostate in a conformal manner (> 96 Gy).
- Dosimetry is determined after insertion of the needles so dosing is much more uniform.
- Treatment with high-dose iridium radiation kills fast-growing tumors more effectively.

69

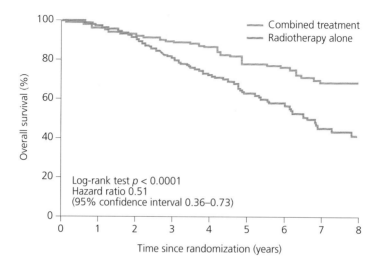

Figure 5.7 Kaplan–Meier estimates of survival for men with high-risk prostate cancer treated with external-beam radiotherapy alone and in combination with hormone therapy for 3 years.

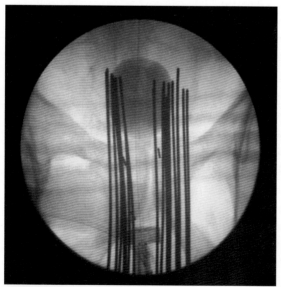

Figure 5.8 An X-ray of a man being treated with high-dose-rate (HDR) brachytherapy. Needles have been placed in the prostate and the balloon in the catheter has been filled with contrast.

High-dose-rate (HDR) brachytherapy can be given as monotherapy or as a prostatic boost in combination with external-beam radiotherapy. The results when used in combination with external-beam radiotherapy for intermediate- and high-risk cancer are quite good. The 10-year disease-free survival rate is approximately 69% and cancer-specific survival is 93%. HDR brachytherapy as monotherapy can be used as an alternative to seed brachytherapy. Although only early results are available, cancer control appears to be equivalent, with possibly fewer side effects with HDR brachytherapy.

Hormonal treatment alone. A full discussion of hormonal therapy is given in Chapter 7. Conventional hormone ablation therapy for locally advanced prostate cancer involves the use of depot LHRH analogs, preceded and accompanied by an antiandrogen for at least 2–6 weeks and sometimes continued thereafter for a period of up to 3 years.

Monotherapy with antiandrogens. Monotherapy with the antiandrogen bicalutamide, 150 mg/day, has been shown in randomized trials to be as effective in controlling locally advanced disease as castration treatment by either orchidectomy or LHRH analog. In addition, a very large, randomized, international trial, with median follow up of 7.4 years, has shown that adjuvant treatment with bicalutamide, 150 mg/day, plus standard therapy for locally advanced prostate cancer (i.e. surgery, radiotherapy or watchful waiting) clearly results in a highly significant reduction in objective progression of 31% when compared with placebo plus standard therapy. A survival benefit of 35% was also observed in men undergoing radiation with adjuvant bicalutamide (Figure 5.9). The advantage of using the antiandrogen option is that sexual interest and function may be preserved (Figure 5.10). Younger patients may often opt for treatment that has a lesser impact on this important aspect of their lives. They should be warned, however, of the possibility of gynecomastia.

Management of local complications

Locally advanced prostate cancer may precipitate any of several urologic emergencies. Acute or chronic urinary retention may require TURP. Care should be taken with this procedure not to induce urinary

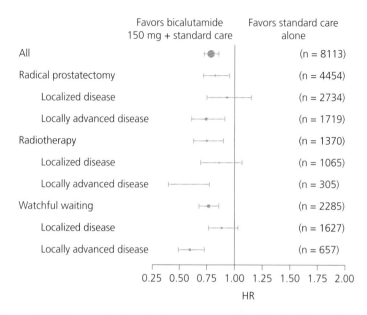

Figure 5.9 A forest plot showing improvements in objective disease-free survival for men randomized to adjuvant bicalutamide, 150 mg/day, plus standard care compared with those receiving placebo plus standard care. Reproduced with permission from McLeod et al. 2006. Copyright Blackwell Publishing. HR, hazard ratio.

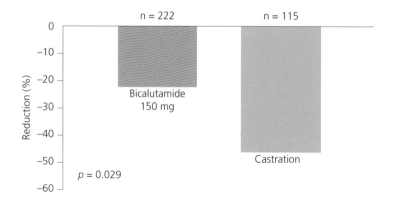

Figure 5.10 Percentage reduction from baseline in sexual interest after 12 months' treatment: bicalutamide, 150 mg, versus castration in M0 patients. Adapted from Iversen P. *Eur Urol* 1999;36(suppl 2):20–6.

incontinence because the normal landmarks can be distorted by the tumor. A period of catheter drainage during androgen ablation, followed by a trial without the catheter, is often indicated. Anuria resulting from bilateral ureteric obstruction, either at the vesico-ureteric junction or at the pelvic brim due to enlarged lymph nodes, may necessitate insertion of nephrostomy tubes or passage of a double-pigtail stent and subsequent external-beam radiotherapy. Bleeding from the tumor may occasionally precipitate hematuria and clot retention, requiring bladder washout and irrigation, and sometimes diathermy or even embolization of bleeding tumor vessels.

An algorithm for the management of men with localized or high-risk prostate cancer is given in Figure 5.11.

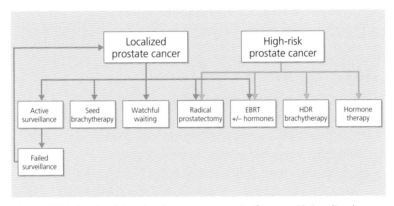

Figure 5.11 An algorithm for the management of men with localized or high-risk prostate cancer. EBRT, external-beam radiotherapy; HDR, high-dose-rate.

Key points – management of localized disease

- The treatment of localized prostate cancer is controversial.
- Radical prostatectomy probably offers the best prospect of long-term cure, but carries the disadvantage of possible sexual dysfunction and incontinence.
- External-beam radiotherapy can be curative, but is associated with possible rectal and bladder complications.
- Brachytherapy is gaining in popularity and can be combined with external-beam radiotherapy in high-risk individuals.

Key points – management of high-risk disease

- Men with high-risk disease have local tumor spread beyond the prostate, or tumor within the prostate but high PSA level or Gleason score.
- Local staging by MRI may be helpful but is subject to inaccuracies.
- Treatment with external-beam radiotherapy and hormonal therapy is more effective than radiotherapy alone.
- A large, international trial confirmed that treatment with the antiandrogen bicalutamide, 150 mg/day, reduced objective progression by 31%.

Key references

Albertsen PC, Hanley JA, Fine J. 20-year outcomes following conservative management of clinically localized prostate cancer. *JAMA* 2005;293:2095–101.

Aus G, Pileblad E, Hugosson J. Cryosurgical ablation of the prostate: 5-year follow-up of a prospective study. *Eur Urol* 2002;42:133–8.

Bacon CG, Giovannucci E, Testa M, Kawachi I. The impact of cancer treatment on quality of life outcomes for patients with localized prostate cancer. *J Urol* 2001;166:1804–10.

Bill-Axelson A, Holmberg L, Ruutu M et al. Radical prostatectomy versus watchful waiting in early prostate cancer. *N Engl J Med* 2005;352:1977–84.

Blasko JC, Mate T, Sylvester JE et al. Brachytherapy for carcinoma of the prostate: techniques, patient selection, and clinical outcomes. *Semin Radiat Oncol* 2002;12:81–94.

Bolla M, Collette L, Blank L et al. Long-term results with immediate androgen suppression and external irradiation in patients with locally advanced prostate cancer (an EORTC study): a phase III randomised trial. *Lancet* 2002; 360:103–6.

Bolla M, van Poppel H, Collette L et al. Postoperative radiotherapy after radical prostatectomy: a randomised controlled trial (EORTC trial 22911). *Lancet* 2005;366:572–8.

Brawer MK. Bicalutamide as immediate therapy either alone or as adjuvant to the standard care of patients with localized or locally advanced prostate cancer: first analysis of the Early Prostate Cancer program. *BJU Int* 2003;91:465–6.

Chawla AK, Thakral HK, Zietman AL, Shipley WU. Salvage radiotherapy after radical prostatectomy for prostate adenocarcinoma: analysis of efficacy and prognostic factors. *Urology* 2002;59:726–31.

D'Amico AV, Chen MH, Renshaw AA et al Androgen suppression and radiation vs radiation alone for prostate cancer: a randomized trial. *JAMA* 2008;299:289–95.

D'Amico AV, Denham JW, Bolla M et al. Short- vs long-term androgen suppression plus external beam radiation therapy and survival in men of advanced age with node-negative high-risk adenocarcinoma of the prostate. *Cancer* 2007;109:2004–10.

D'Amico AV, Whittington R, Malkowicz SB et al. Predicting prostate specific antigen outcome preoperatively in the prostate specific antigen era. *J Urol* 2001;166:2185–8.

Davis JW, Kuban DA, Lynch DF, Schellhammer PF. Quality of life after treatment for localized prostate cancer: differences based on treatment modality. *J Urol* 2001; 166:947–52.

Gleave ME, Goldenberg L, Jones EC. Biochemical and pathological effects of 8 months of neoadjuvant androgen withdrawal therapy before radical prostatectomy in patients with clinically confined prostate cancer. *J Urol* 1996;155:213–19.

Graefen M, Karakiewicz PI, Cagiannos I et al. International validation of a preoperative nomogram for prostate cancer recurrence after radical prostatectomy. *J Clin Oncol* 2002;20:3206–12.

Hellerstedt BA, Pienta KJ. The current state of hormonal therapy for prostate cancer. *CA Cancer J Clin* 2002;52:154–79.

Holmberg L, Bill-Axelson A, Helgesen F et al. A randomized trial comparing radical prostatectomy with watchful waiting in early prostate cancer. *N Engl J Med* 2002;347:781–9.

Iversen P. Antiandrogen monotherapy: indications and results. *Urology* 2002;60(suppl 1):64–71.

Iversen P, Tyrrell CJ, Kaisary AM *et al.* Bicalutamide monotherapy compared with castration in patients with nonmetastaic locally advanced prostate cancer: 6.3 years of follow-up. *J Urol* 2000;164:1579–82.

Klein EA, Kupelian PA, Dreicer R et al. Locally advanced prostate cancer. *Curr Treat Options Oncol* 2001;2:403–11.

Klotz LH. Low-risk prostate cancer can and should often be managed with active surveillance and selective delayed intervention. *Nat Clin Pract Urol* 2008;5:2–3.

Klotz, L. Active surveillance with selective delayed intervention is the way to manage 'good-risk' prostate cancer. *Nat Clin Pract Urol* 2005;2:136–42.

Korb LJ, Brawer MK. Modern brachytherapy for localized prostate cancers: the Northwest Hospital (Seattle) experience. *Rev Urol* 2001;3:51–61.

Kupelian PA, Elshaikh M, Reddy CA, Zippe C, Klein EA. Comparison of the efficacy of local therapies for localized prostate cancer in the prostate-specific antigen era: a large single-institution experience with radical prostatectomy and external-beam radiotherapy. *J Clin Oncol* 2002;20:3376–85.

Lu-Yao GL, Yao SL. Population-based study of long-term survival in patients with clinically localised prostate cancer. *Lancet* 1997;349: 906–10.

Mayer R, Pummer K, Quehenberger F et al. Postprostatectomy radiotherapy for high-risk prostate cancer. *Urology* 2002;59:732–9.

McLeod DG, Iversen P, See WA *et al.* Bicalutamide 150mg plus standard care vs standard care alone for early prostate cancer. *BJU Int* 2006;97:247–54.

Onik G. Image-guided prostate cryosurgery: state of the art. *Cancer Control* 2001;8:522–31.

Pilepich MV, Sause WF, Shipley WU et al. Androgen deprivation with radiation therapy compared with radiation therapy alone for locally advanced prostatic carcinoma: a randomized comparative trial of the Radiation Therapy Oncology Group. *Urology* 1995;45:616–23.

Pilepich MV, Winter K, John MJ et al. Phase III radiation therapy oncology group (RTOG) trial 86-10 of androgen deprivation adjuvant to definitive radiotherapy in locally advanced carcinoma of the prostate. *Int J Radiat Oncol Biol Phys* 2001;50:1243–52.

Pollack A, Zagars GK, Starkschall G et al. Prostate cancer radiation dose response: results of the M. D. Anderson phase III randomized trial. *Int J Radiat Oncol Biol Phys* 2002; 53:1097–105.

Pound CR, Partin AW, Eisenberger MA. Natural history of progression after PSA elevation following radical prostatectomy. *JAMA* 1999;281:1591–7.

Pound CW, Brawer MK, Partin AW. Evaluation and treatment of men with biochemical prostate specific antigen recurrence following definitive therapy for clinically localized prostate cancer. *Rev Urol* 2001;3:72–84.

Ragde H, Elgamal AA, Snow PB et al. Ten-year disease free survival after transperineal sonography-guided iodine-125 brachytherapy with or without 45-gray external beam irradiation in the treatment of patients with clinically localized, low to high Gleason grade prostate carcinoma. *Cancer* 1998;83: 989–1001.

Salomon L, Levrel O, de la Taille A et al. Radical prostatectomy by the retropubic, perineal and laparoscopic approach: 12 years of experience in one center. *Eur Urol* 2002;42:104–10.

Sharkey J, Cantor A, Solc Z et al. Brachytherapy versus radical prostatectomy in patients with clinically localized prostate cancer. *Curr Urol Rep* 2002;3:250–7.

Soffen EM, Hanks GE, Hwang CC et al. Conformal static field therapy for low grade prostate cancer with rigid immobilization. *Int J Radiat Biol Phys* 1992;24:485–8.

Soloway MS, Sharifi R, Wajsman Z et al. Randomized prospective study comparing radical prostatectomy alone versus radical prostatectomy preceded by androgen blockade in clinical stage B2 (T2bNxM0) prostate cancer. The Lupron Depot Neoadjuvant Prostate Cancer Study Group. *J Urol* 1995;154:424–8.

Stanford JL, Feng Z, Hamilton AS et al. Urinary and sexual function after radical prostatectomy for clinically localized prostate cancer: the Prostate Cancer Outcomes Study. *JAMA* 2000;283:354–60.

Stone NN, Stock RG. Permanent seed implantation for localized adenocarcinoma of the prostate. *Curr Urol Rep* 2002;3:201–6.

Tewari A, Peabody J, Sarle R et al. Technique of da Vinci robot-assisted anatomic radical prostatectomy. *Urology* 2002;60:569–72.

Thompson IM, Tangen CM, Paradelo J et al. Adjuvant radiotherapy for pathologically advanced prostate cancer: a randomized clinical trial. *JAMA* 2006; 296:2329–35.

Uchida T, Ohkusa H, Yamashita H et al. Five years experience of transrectal high-intensity focused ultrasound using the Sonablate device in the treatment of localized prostate cancer. *Int J Urol* 2006;13:228–33.

Vargas C, Martinez A, Galalae R et al. High-dose radiation employing external beam radiotherapy and high-dose rate brachytherapy with and without neoadjuvant androgen deprivation for prostate cancer patients with intermediate- and high-risk features. *Prostate Cancer Prostatic Dis* 2006;9:245–53.

Walsh PC. Surgery and the reduction of mortality from prostate cancer. *N Engl J Med* 2002;347:839–40.

Wilt TJ. Clarifying uncertainty regarding detection and treatment of early-stage prostate cancer. *Semin Urol Oncol* 2002;20:10–17.

Wilt TJ, Brawer MK. The prostate cancer intervention versus observation trial (PIVOT). *Oncology* 1997;11:1133–43.

Wirth M, Tyrrell C, Wallace M et al. Bicalutamide (Casodex) 150 mg as immediate therapy in patients with localized or locally advanced prostate cancer significantly reduces the risk of disease progression. *Urology* 2001;58:146–51.

Zelefsky MJ, Leibel SA, Gaudin PB et al. Dose escalation with three-dimensional conformal radiation therapy affects the outcome in prostate cancer. *Int J Radiat Oncol Biol Phys* 1998;41:491–500.

Zisman A, Pantuck AJ, Cohen JK, Belldegrun AS. Prostate cryoablation using direct transperineal placement of ultrathin probes through a 17-gauge brachytherapy template-technique and preliminary results. *Urology* 2001;58:988–93.

Following treatment be it by surgery or radiotherapy, recurrence is usually first manifest as a lone rise in the PSA. DRE, CT scan or MRI and bone scan are the next steps, but unless the PSA level is very high, these tests do not usually reveal a site. The ProstaScint scan, which is based on a radioimmunoassay for prostate-specific membrane antigen, may reveal sites of metastases not identified by other means but not infrequently gives false-positive results; the investigation is still regarded as experimental.

Recurrence following prostatectomy

Of men undergoing radical prostatectomy, 15–46% suffer cancer recurrence in the form of a postoperative rise in PSA. Following prostatectomy, the PSA level should fall to below 0.1 ng/mL. The recommendations for cut-off values to indicate cancer recurrence vary from 0.2 ng/mL to 0.5 ng/mL. If the PSA level does not fall to below this level within 6 weeks postoperatively, the presence of systemic disease should be considered.

Cancer recurrence is confirmed once a patient has a PSA level above the cut-off and it is rising, but time to metastasis and death can be quite variable. On average, a patient with a PSA recurrence will develop metastases over a median of 8 years, with a further 5 years to death from prostate cancer. This is, however, very variable, and a number of factors determine how fast the cancer recurrence will actually progress:

- time to recurrence, as a shorter time to recurrence results in faster progression of disease
- time it takes for the PSA to double, as a doubling time of less than 3 months is associated with shorter time to metastases and death
- Gleason score.

When cancer recurs by PSA level only, it is not known whether the recurrence is local (in the prostate bed) or systemic (metastases). A number of factors can also help with estimation of the likelihood of local versus systemic disease. Table 6.1 outlines the major factors.

TABLE 6.1

PSA and pathology variables that predict local or systemic recurrence following radical prostatectomy

Variable	Local recurrence	Systemic recurrence
Gleason score	≤ 7	> 7
Lymph node invasion	No	Yes
PSA doubling time	> 12 months	< 3 months
Seminal vesicle involvement	No	Yes
Time to PSA recurrence	> 1 year	< 1 year

The management of PSA recurrence consists of a number of choices. These include watchful waiting, salvage radiotherapy or hormonal therapy.

Watchful waiting is ideal for the man with a limited life-expectancy and/or lower probability of disease progression based on the earlier criteria. It should be remembered that, in the average patient, metastases do not develop until 8 years after a PSA rise is detected, with death 13 years later.

Salvage radiotherapy is a treatment given to men who have a high likelihood of residual cancer in the prostatic bed. The best results are in those men who have Gleason score of 7 or less, pre-radiotherapy PSA below 2.0 ng/mL, positive surgical margins, and a PSA doubling time of more than 10 months. The efficacy of salvage radiation is improving, with 60–90% of men achieving undetectable PSA levels. Side effects include possible loss of erectile function, bladder neck contracture and proctitis.

Hormonal therapy is reserved for men who have progressive PSA rises and are unlikely to harbor isolated local recurrence. In these men with presumed systemic disease, the timing of when to start hormonal therapy is controversial. There is evidence that hormonal therapy started early in patients with an asymptomatic increase in PSA results in delayed development of bone metastases, but it has not been shown to improve survival. For more information on hormone therapy, see Chapter 7.

Recurrence following radiation therapy

The definition of recurrence after radiation treatment is less straightforward than that after surgery. Following radiation, the PSA falls slowly over 12–24 months to a nadir at detectable levels, usually below 1.0 ng/mL. In addition, approximately 30% of men have a transient rise (a 'bounce'). To complicate matters further, adjuvant hormonal therapy is often used and suppresses PSA, but once it is stopped the PSA slowly rises as the testosterone levels rise.

Currently, recurrence after radiation therapy is defined as PSA 2 ng/mL above the nadir level. The natural history of PSA recurrence is not as clear in patients who have had radiation therapy as in those who have had surgery. PSA doubling time is clearly the best predictor of metastatic disease, and in fact a PSA doubling time of less than 3 months is also associated with a higher risk of death.

Once a PSA recurrence has been defined, further investigations depend on the individual's circumstances and expectations and involve determining whether the cancer is present in the prostate, whether it is systemic, or both. ProstaScint imaging can be used in addition to the staging imaging of a bone scan and CT or MRI, though it is still considered experimental. A prostate re-biopsy can be performed if treatment for local disease is being considered, but the result is often negative.

Options for treatment of recurrence after radiation are multiple. Watchful waiting can be offered to men who have limited life-expectancy and/or slow progression of their cancer. Men who are likely to have cancer limited to the prostate have a number of options that include salvage prostatectomy, which is more difficult than it is in men who have not had radiation and also has a significantly higher incidence of side effects. Cryotherapy and HIFU therapy are also options and have been outlined previously. Hormonal therapy is usually reserved for men who are unlikely to have localized disease only and have progressive disease.

As with hormone therapy after prostatectomy, the timing of hormone therapy for recurrence after radiation therapy is still controversial.

Key points – managing recurrence after initial therapy

- PSA level should fall to below 0.1 ng/mL following prostatectomy.
- Recurrence after prostatectomy is generally defined as PSA above 0.2 ng/mL.
- Recurrence after radiation therapy is defined as PSA 2 ng/mL above the nadir level.
- For the average patient, metastases do not develop until 8 years after a PSA rise is detected, so watchful waiting is an appropriate option for some men with recurrence.
- More evidence is needed from clinical trials to inform us of the best treatment options in this situation.

Key references

Bianco FJ Jr, Scardino PT, Stephenson AJ et al. Long-term oncologic results of salvage radical prostatectomy for locally recurrent prostate cancer after radiotherapy. *Int J Radiat Oncol Biol Phys* 2005;62:448–53.

D'Amico AV, Moul J, Carroll PR et al. Prostate specific antigen doubling time as a surrogate end point for prostate cancer specific mortality following radical prostatectomy or radiation therapy. *J Urol* 2004;172:S42–6.

Freedland SJ, Humphreys EB, Mangold LA et al. Risk of prostate cancer-specific mortality following biochemical recurrence after radical prostatectomy. *JAMA* 2005;294: 433–9.

Lee WR, Hanks GE, Hanlon A. Increasing prostate-specific antigen profile following definitive radiation therapy for localized prostate cancer: clinical observations. *J Clin Oncol* 1997;15:230–8.

Pound CR, Partin AW, Eisenberger MA et al. Natural history of progression after PSA elevation following radical prostatectomy. *JAMA* 1999;281: 1591–7.

Roach M 3rd, Hanks G, Thames H Jr et al. Defining biochemical failure following radiotherapy with or without hormonal therapy in men with clinically localized prostate cancer: recommendations of the RTOG-ASTRO Phoenix Consensus Conference. *Int J Radiat Oncol Biol Phys* 2006;65:965–74.

Stephenson AJ, Shariat SF, Zelefsky MJ et al. Salvage radiotherapy for recurrent prostate cancer after radical prostatectomy. *JAMA* 2004;291:1325–32.

Thompson IM, Tangen CM, Paradelo J et al. Adjuvant radiotherapy for pathological T3N0M0 prostate cancer significantly reduces risk of metastases and improves survival: long-term followup of a randomized clinical trial. *J Urol* 2009;181:956–62.

Trock BJ. Han M, Freedland SJ et al. Prostate-specific survival following salvage radiotherapy vs observation in men with biochemical recurrence after radical prostatectomy. *JAMA* 2008;299:2760–9.

Van der Kwast TH, Bolla M, Van Poppel H et al. Identification of patients with prostate cancer who benefit from immediate postoperative radiotherapy: EORTC 22911. *J Clin Oncol* 2007;25:4178–86.

Although there is an increasing trend towards earlier detection of prostate cancer, many men throughout the world still present with metastatic disease. In countries where PSA testing is not widely used, around 30% of patients present with localized disease, 40% with locally advanced disease and the remaining 30% with metastases. In contrast to localized or locally advanced disease, metastatic prostate cancer is associated with high mortality – approximately 70% within 5 years. Androgen deprivation, which has become the mainstay of treatment, effectively reduces intraprostatic DHT concentration by over 80%, resulting in reduced androgen-receptor stimulation and increased prostate cancer apoptosis (Table 7.1). Androgen deprivation can be achieved by orchidectomy or treatment with LHRH analogs, and the value of adding an antiandrogen (maximal androgen blockade) is still debated. Pure LHRH antagonists are currently under investigation, but are not yet approved by regulatory authorities.

Orchidectomy

Bilateral orchidectomy or bilateral subcapsular orchidectomy is performed through a midline scrotal incision (Figure 7.1) under local, regional or light general anesthesia. The procedure is simple and is associated with little morbidity. The principal adverse events that may occur after orchidectomy are local complications such as hematoma and

TABLE 7.1

Treatment options for metastatic prostate cancer

- Androgen deprivation
  - orchidectomy
  - LHRH analogs
- Maximal androgen blockade
- Intermittent androgen blockade

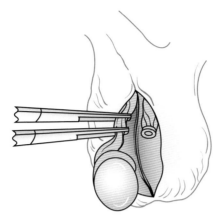

Figure 7.1 Bilateral orchidectomy is generally performed via a midline scrotal incision.

wound infections, together with general complications of androgen deprivation such as loss of libido, erectile dysfunction and hot flashes (Table 7.2). Clinical responses (decreased bone pain and reduced PSA concentration) are obtained in more than 75% of patients. Because of the psychological and cosmetic impact of orchidectomy, however, most patients and their partners prefer reversible non-surgical treatment with LHRH analogs.

TABLE 7.2

Side effects of androgen-deprivation therapy

- Hot flashes
- Decreased libido
- Lethargy
- Cognitive decline
- Mood changes
- Osteoporosis
- Weight gain
- Loss of muscle mass

LHRH analogs

LHRH analogs, such as goserelin acetate, buserelin and leuprolide, are highly potent LHRH agonists (superagonists). After administration, there is a transient initial increase in luteinizing hormone (LH) secretion, and hence in testosterone secretion; this is followed by desensitization (downregulation), resulting in a fall in LH and testosterone secretion (Figure 7.2). These agents can be delivered via 1-, 3- or 6-monthly depot preparations administered subcutaneously or intramuscularly. A potential side effect is tumor 'flare', which 8–32% of patients experience as a result of the initial transient increase (140–170%) in testosterone. This may result in increased bone pain or worsening of symptoms of bladder outflow obstruction; spinal metastases may also be stimulated, increasing a risk of spinal cord compression. Tumor flare can be avoided by prior and concomitant administration of an antiandrogen during the

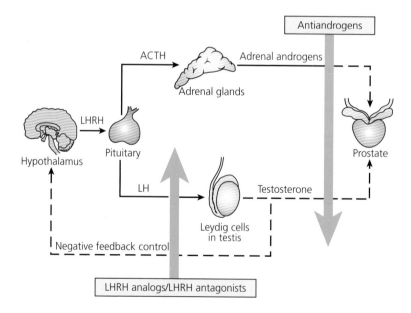

Figure 7.2 LHRH analogs inhibit pituitary LH secretion, and thus reduce testicular androgen secretion. Antiandrogens act peripherally to block testosterone action on androgen receptors. ACTH, adrenocorticotropic hormone.

first 6 weeks of treatment. Comparative trials have shown that the response rates obtained with LHRH analogs are equivalent to those obtained after orchidectomy in terms of time to progression and overall survival.

LHRH antagonists

Recently, pure LHRH (or GnRH) antagonists have been developed and evaluated. These peptides inhibit LHRH release without causing the initial stimulation seen with LHRH analogs by blocking pituitary receptors and thus they are not associated with a surge in testosterone (flare). Abarelix and degarelix, both LHRH antagonists, have shown positive clinical results in controlled clinical studies involving men with hormone-sensitive prostate cancer (Figure 7.3). A rapid reduction in testosterone without a flare was achieved with both antagonists, compared with the significant flare resulting from the administration of an LHRH analog. PSA rapidly decreased in both cases and this effect was maintained in the long term with both agents. Abarelix has been associated with occasional hypersensitivity. LHRH antagonists may be beneficial for patients with bony metastases or bladder neck obstruction where tumor control without testosterone surge is important. An additional potential benefit could be in men receiving intermittent hormonal therapy, in whom the rapid return to LHRH receptor function following withdrawal of the drug results in an accompanying rapid return of testosterone.

Antiandrogens

Antiandrogens are taken in tablet form and do not alter the levels of circulating androgens. Instead, they inhibit the androgen receptor where testosterone or DHT binds. There are two classes of these drugs. The steroidal antiandrogens, e.g. cyproterone acetate, also have a central testosterone-lowering effect and can be taken as monotherapy instead of castration. The non-steroidal antiandrogens inhibit the androgen receptor only and should not be taken as monotherapy for metastatic disease as the results are inferior to those achieved with LHRH analogs.

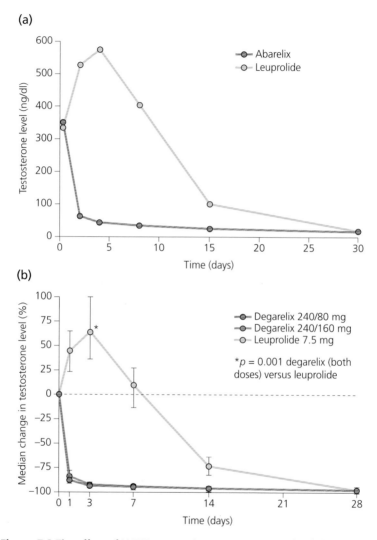

Figure 7.3 The effect of LHRH antagonists on testosterone level. (a) Results from a phase III study comparing abarelix depot with leuprolide depot in men with prostate cancer (for testosterone in nmol/l, multiply by 0.0347). (b) Degarelix at a starting dose of 240 mg followed by a monthly maintenance dose of either 80 mg or 160 mg reduced serum testosterone level more rapidly than leuprolide at the standard monthly dose of 7.5 mg. This phase III trial involved 610 men with prostate cancer (any stage). Reproduced with permission from Klotz et al. 2008.

Maximal androgen blockade

Although both orchidectomy and LHRH treatment produce dramatic initial responses in 70–80% of men, remission is not usually maintained in the long term. Androgen-independent cancer cell clones are selected out, so the mean time to tumor progression is less than 18 months and the mean overall survival time is approximately 28–36 months. One factor that may contribute to this poor prognosis is persistent adrenal androgen secretion; there is evidence that adrenal androgens account for up to 15–20% of total androgen concentrations within the prostate. This has led to the concept of maximal androgen blockade, in which androgen deprivation by orchidectomy or LHRH treatment is accompanied by treatment with an antiandrogen to block the effects of adrenal androgens in the prostate.

Maximal androgen blockade with a combination of an LHRH analog and an antiandrogen has been shown in several trials to offer improved survival compared with either LHRH analog treatment alone or orchidectomy. However, other trials have failed to show significant improvements in tumor progression and survival, and a meta-analysis of all studies demonstrated no advantage for combined therapy. This discrepancy may arise from steroidal and non-steroidal antiandrogens being evaluated together. A subgroup analysis of combination treatment with non-steroidal antiandrogens only did show a small survival advantage – 2.9% – for combination therapy compared with monotherapy (Figure 7.4). In addition, it appears that maximal androgen blockade may offer a slight advantage over monotherapy, at least in a subgroup of patients with good performance status (i.e. those who are generally well in themselves) and a relatively restricted metastatic burden. Such treatment should, therefore, be considered in younger and fitter patients who are most likely to die from prostate cancer itself rather than from some comorbid condition. However, the relatively modest benefits need to be weighed against the costs and the small but significant incidence in side effects from the antiandrogens.

The timing of hormonal therapy has been the subject of vigorous debate. The evidence now seems to favor earlier therapy rather than waiting for symptoms. This evidence includes a re-analysis of the cooperative studies (USA) in which men receiving 1 mg of

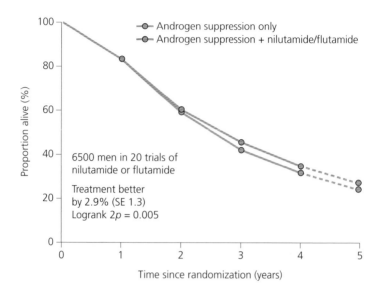

Figure 7.4 Maximal androgen blockade with non-steroidal antiandrogens improves survival by 2.9% when compared with LHRH analog alone. Reproduced, with permission from the Prostate Cancer Trialists' Collaborative Group. Copyright Elsevier 2000.

diethylstilbestrol (DES) had a survival advantage. The Medical Research Council (UK) study showed that men with locally advanced or metastatic disease treated with castration at the time of diagnosis had better outcomes than those receiving deferred therapy (Figure 7.5; Table 7.3), and a US trial reported by Messing et al. found that men with pelvic lymph node metastases treated with delayed hormonal therapy had a sevenfold increase in death from prostate cancer compared with those who had immediate androgen ablation therapy. It is clear that early initiation of hormone therapy in men with locally advanced or metastatic disease improves survival and decreases complications. It is not yet clear how early we should start hormone therapy in men who have rising PSA following primary treatment with surgery or radiotherapy in the absence of demonstrable metastases, even though it is expected that the rising PSA is from metastases. It should be

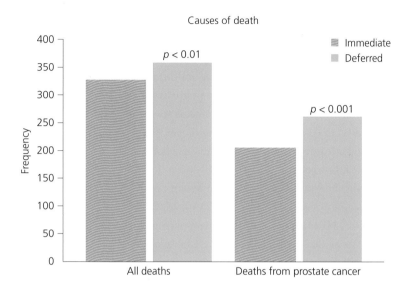

Causes of death

Figure 7.5 Immediate hormonal therapy versus deferred treatment for advanced prostate cancer. Adapted from the Medical Research Council Prostate Cancer Working Party Investigators Group 1997.

TABLE 7.3

Prostate-cancer-related complications in men with locally advanced or metastatic disease randomized to immediate or delayed hormone therapy*

	Immediate hormone therapy (n = 469)	Delayed hormone therapy (n = 465)
Pathological fracture	11	21
Cord compression	9	23
Ureteric obstruction	33	55
Development of extraskeletal metastases	37	55

*Adapted from the Medical Research Council Prostate Cancer Working Party Investigators Group 1997.

borne in mind, however, that earlier treatment with hormonal therapy increases the risk of side effects such as osteoporosis.

Intermittent hormonal therapy

It has been suggested that continuous androgen ablation therapy may, in fact, increase the rate of progression of prostate cancer to an androgen-independent state (see Chapter 8). For this reason, attention is currently focused on the use of intermittent hormonal therapy, which also has the potential advantage of decreasing the side effects of therapy. In this approach, hormone therapy is initially given for approximately 9 months. Intermittent therapy becomes an option for men in whom there is a response to therapy with PSA levels becoming normalized, and their LHRH analog therapy is temporarily discontinued.

Hormone therapy is resumed when the serum PSA concentration returns to pretreatment levels in patients with a PSA at diagnosis below 20 ng/mL, or when PSA increases to more than 20 ng/mL in patients with an initial PSA above this. Such a regimen allows serum testosterone to return to normal, thereby stimulating atrophic cells and rendering them more sensitive to androgen ablation (Figure 7.6). The use of a pure LHRH antagonist, which blocks the receptor without initial stimulation, could be advantageous in this setting owing to the absence of flare and potentially a more rapid restoration of testosterone level after cessation of therapy. In some studies of intermittent hormonal therapy, up to five treatment cycles have been given before evidence of androgen independence has appeared, and during this time men have spent approximately 50% of the time off therapy. Randomized trials of intermittent androgen therapy are currently being undertaken and, until these results are available, the approach should be regarded as investigational. Non-randomized studies suggest that patients on intermittent therapy are not suffering disease progression any faster than those receiving continuous androgen suppression, and they enjoy improvements in their quality of life.

Spinal cord compression and pathological fractures

Sudden onset of low back pain and weakness in the lower limbs, with or without voiding difficulty, in a patient with metastatic prostate cancer should be considered to be a urologic/neurosurgical emergency. Spinal cord compression, due to pathological fracture or collapse of the lumbar vertebrae, is the most common reason for these symptoms (Figure 7.7). The diagnosis may be confirmed by urgent spinal MRI. Early

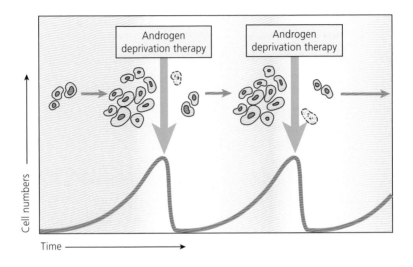

Figure 7.6 Intermittent androgen ablation therapy allows serum testosterone to return periodically to normal, thereby stimulating atrophic cells and rendering them sensitive to subsequent androgen ablation.

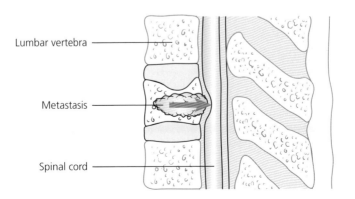

Figure 7.7 Spinal cord compression as a result of a spinal metastasis.

neurosurgical decompression is often advised, usually followed by external-beam radiotherapy and corticosteroids.

Pathological fractures caused by prostate cancer metastases may occur elsewhere, for example in the femur or humerus. Fixation by an orthopedic specialist is often required and should usually be followed by external-beam radiotherapy and androgen ablation.

Key points – management of metastatic disease

- Metastatic prostate cancer is characterized by a positive bone scan and/or the presence of soft tissue metastases.
- PSA values are usually high, often above 50 ng/mL.
- Treatment is usually by androgen ablation.
- An LHRH analog preceded and then accompanied by an antiandrogen is the most frequently employed treatment strategy.
- Responses in terms of PSA reduction and clinical improvement are seen in more than 80% of patients.
- Eventually, however, androgen-insensitive cell clones develop and the PSA level begins to rise.

Key references

Crawford ED, Eisenberger MA, McLeod DG et al. A controlled trial of leuprolide with and without flutamide in prostatic carcinoma. N Engl J Med 1989;321:419–24.

Denis LD, Carneiro de Moura JL, Bono A et al. Goserelin acetate and flutamide versus bilateral orchidectomy: a phase III EORTC trial (30853). Urology 1993;42: 119–29.

Errejon A, Crawford ED. Monotherapy versus combined androgen blockade in patients with advanced prostate cancer. Cancer 2002;95:209–10.

Holmes-Walker DJ, Woo H, Gurney H et al. Maintaining bone health in patients with prostate cancer. Med J Aust 2006;184:176–9.

Janknegt RA, Abbou CC, Bartoletti R et al. Orchidectomy and nilutamide or placebo as treatment of metastatic prostatic cancer in a multinational double-blind randomised trial. *J Urol* 1993;149: 77–83.

Klotz L, Boccon-Gibod L, Shore ND et al. The efficacy and safety of degarelix: a 12 month, comparative randomised, open-label, parallel-group phase III study in prostate cancer patients. *BJU Int* 2008;102:1531–8.

Maximum androgen blockade in advanced prostate cancer: an overview of the randomised trials. Prostate Cancer Trialists' Collaborative Group. *Lancet* 2000;355:1491–8.

Medical Research Council Prostate Cancer Working Party Investigators Group. Immediate versus deferred treatment for advanced prostate cancer: initial results of the MRC Trial. *Br J Urol* 1997;79:235–46.

Messing EM, Manola J, Yao J et al. Immediate versus deferred androgen deprivation treatment in patients with node-positive prostate cancer after radical prostatectomy and pelvic lymphadenectomy. *Lancet Oncol* 2006;7:472–9.

Mittan D, Lee S, Miller E et al. Bone loss following hypogonadism in men with prostate cancer treated with GnRH analogs. *J Clin Endocrinol Metab* 2002;87:3656–61.

Prostate Cancer Trialists Collaborative Group. Maximum androgen blockade in advanced prostate cancer: an overview of 22 randomized trials with 3283 deaths in 5710 patients. *Lancet* 1995;346: 265–9.

Schellhammer PF, Sharifi R, Block NL. Clinical benefits of bicalutamide compared with flutamide in combined androgen blockade for patients with advanced prostatic carcinoma: final report of a double-blind, randomized multicentre trial. *Urology* 1997;50:330–6.

Trachtenberg J, Gittleman M, Steidle C et al. A phase 3, multicenter, open label, randomized study of abarelix versus leuprolide plus daily antiandrogen in men with prostate cancer. *J Urol* 2002;167:1670–4.

Tyrrell CJ, Denis L, Newling D et al. Casodex™ 10–200 mg daily used as monotherapy for the treatment of patients with advanced prostate cancer. An overview of the efficacy, tolerability and pharmacokinetics from three phase II dose-ranging studies. Casodex Study Group. *Eur Urol* 1998;33:39–53.

8 Management of androgen-independent disease

In most cases, advanced prostate cancers treated with any form of androgen deprivation eventually begin to progress, a phenomenon known as 'hormone-refractory' or 'androgen-independent' disease. This is probably due to either clonal selection of androgen-independent cell lines (Figure 8.1) or increased ligand-independent activation of androgen receptors. Thus, an increase in PSA level after initially successful androgen deprivation almost inevitably indicates impending clinical progression. This group is, however, quite heterogeneous, including men with PSA rises only and no demonstrable metastases, and men who have many bone and visceral metastases, pain and poor functional status; survival can range from only a few months to 4 years. Historically, therapy had little impact beyond modest palliation; however, treatments that may delay the progression of symptoms and reduce serum PSA are becoming available (Table 8.1).

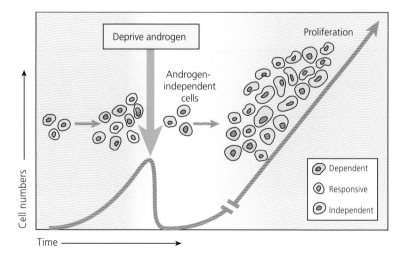

Figure 8.1 Hormone escape results from the selection of androgen-independent cell lines.

TABLE 8.1

Treatments for androgen-independent prostate cancer

- Antiandrogen manipulation
- Adrenal androgen synthesis inhibitors
- Estrogen
- Cytotoxic chemotherapy
- Radiotherapy
- Bisphosphonates
- Clinical trial of experimental agent(s)

Antiandrogen manipulation

When the serum PSA level rises after a period of androgen-deprivation therapy alone, an initial move may be to add an antiandrogen to the treatment. This may have an effect in reducing PSA, but after some time the PSA will start to rise again. At this time withdrawal of the antiandrogen treatment may also result in a favorable PSA response (in approximately 40% of men). This phenomenon (which also occurs in breast cancer treated with antiestrogens) has been ascribed to a mutation of androgen receptors in malignant tissue that renders the antiandrogen an agonist rather than an antagonist in effect. This response may last for a few months, after which the PSA will start to rise again. As long as the patient is asymptomatic, the addition and withdrawal of different antiandrogens can be continued for two to three cycles, as prior antiandrogen administration does not appear to diminish the response to further antiandrogen administration.

In addition to antiandrogens, research has shown that antiandrogen withdrawal followed by inhibitors of adrenal androgen synthesis, such as aminoglutethimide or ketoconazole, results in good reductions in PSA levels. However, adrenal androgen synthesis inhibitors are very toxic and not well tolerated, so this is not a usual treatment option.

Estrogen

Estrogen treatment may benefit some men with androgen-independent prostate cancer. Such treatment appears to have two effects:

97

- inhibition of pituitary gonadotropin secretion
- direct cytotoxic effect on the tumor.

The synthetic estrogen DES has been used in prostate cancer, but its use as first-line therapy is limited by side effects such as gynecomastia, deep-vein thrombosis and other cardiovascular complications. Combination of DES with aspirin or coumadin may reduce the thrombotic and cardiovascular toxicity that can be hazardous in men of this age, but patients should be alerted to the risks.

Cytotoxic therapy

Mitoxantrone and prednisone was the first chemotherapy combination to be tested in a randomized fashion in advanced prostate cancer. The trial showed that this combination was very well tolerated and reduced PSA levels significantly. The combination has been shown to more than double the time of palliation response when compared with prednisone alone and to improve the quality of life of men with androgen-independent prostate cancer. In asymptomatic men with metastases it also prolonged the time to disease progression. This combination has not, however, been shown to increase survival time.

Docetaxel, another chemotherapy agent, which is a member of the taxoid family, induces apoptosis in cells through microtubule depolymerization. It has been tested in a randomized trial against mitoxantrone and prednisone in men with androgen-independent prostate cancer. The results of this study (TAX-327) were reported in 2004 and showed docetaxel, given in a 3-week schedule, to be superior to mitoxantrone/prednisone in terms of decreasing disease progression, PSA response and improving pain. In addition, docetaxel significantly improved survival from a median of 16.4 months for mitoxantrone/prednisone to 18.9 months for 3-weekly docetaxel, which correlates to a 24% relative reduction in death (Figure 8.2). Docetaxel was also administered weekly in one of the arms of this study and this did not show any significant survival advantage over mitoxantrone/prednisone when given in this manner. The side effects associated with docetaxel include neutropenia, skin reactions and gastrointestinal problems. In the trial described, the incidence of these

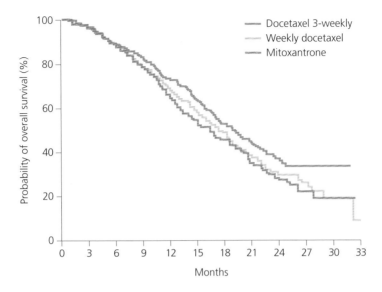

Figure 8.2 Kaplan–Meier estimates of overall survival in the three arms of the TAX-327 study. Docetaxel, 3-weekly, improved survival by 24% (hazard ratio 0.76) compared with mitoxantrone and prednisone. Reproduced, with permission, from Tannock et al. 2004. Copyright © 2004 Massachusetts Medical Society. All rights reserved.

side effects was higher in the group receiving docetaxel than in the group receiving the mitoxantrone/prednisone combination. However, docetaxel is generally well tolerated, and overall quality of life was better for the men who had received docetaxel compared with those who had received mitoxantrone/prednisone.

Estramustine phosphate combines a nitrogen mustard agent with phosphorylated estradiol and in combination with docetaxel it has been compared with mitoxantrone/prednisone. The combination showed a survival benefit, PSA response and time to progression delay similar to those achieved with docetaxel alone in TAX-327 (Figure 8.3). Unfortunately, this combination is quite toxic, predominately because of cardiovascular and thromboembolic events. As the survival benefit was similar to that achieved with docetaxel alone, it is unlikely this combination will be commonly used.

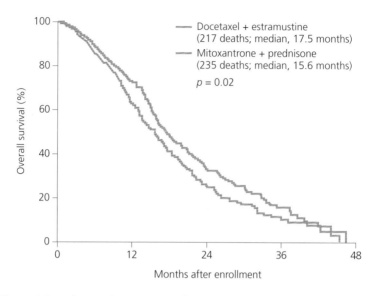

Figure 8.3 Kaplan–Meier estimates of overall survival in the SWOG 99-16 study. Treatment with docetaxel and estramustine improved survival by more than 2 months compared with mitoxantrone and prednisone. Reproduced, with permission, from Petrylak et al. 2004. Copyright © 2004 Massachusetts Medical Society. All rights reserved.

Management of bone metastases

Bone pain is one of the most intractable problems associated with androgen-independent prostate cancer, and conventional analgesics may not always provide relief.

Palliative radiotherapy. Men with hormone-naïve disease will initially be managed by androgen-deprivation therapy. But some men will not get full pain resolution or may have painful bone metastases in the setting of androgen-independent prostate cancer. For these men, focal external-beam radiotherapy is a well-established treatment, and up to 80% of treated men will experience rapid improvement in pain. Treatment can be given as a single fraction or as multiple fractions over 2–3 weeks. There are very few side effects associated with this type of irradiation.

Wide-field radiation may also be useful in patients with intractable diffuse pain. This treatment can delay the progression of existing disease as well as slow the occurrence of new disease, but it produces side effects such as pneumonitis, cataracts, nausea, vomiting and diarrhea in approximately 35% of patients, and severe, sometimes irreversible, hematological effects in 9%.

Systemic radionuclide therapy is a means of targeting multiple painful bone metastases by intravenously administering a radionuclide (such as samarium-153) complexed to bone-avid molecules such as ethylenediamine-tetra (methylene phosphonic acid) (EDTMP), or radionuclides that have a natural affinity to metabolically active bone, such as strontium-89. After administration of samarium-153, 65–80% of patients report relief from pain and symptoms within 1 week. The average duration of response is 2–3 months. The major toxicity is myelosuppresion, which can last a number of months – white blood cell count and platelet levels should be monitored before and after therapy.

Bisphosphonates. Some patients benefit symptomatically from treatment with bisphosphonates, which suppress bone resorption and demineralization. A study involving over 600 patients with androgen-independent prostate cancer compared zoledronic acid, given as an intravenous infusion over 15 minutes every 3 weeks, with placebo. There was a significant reduction in the number of patients with skeletal-related events, and the first such event was significantly delayed in the bisphosphonate-treated arm (Figure 8.4). It would, however, require ten men to be treated to save one from a skeletal-related event. Side effects include renal deterioration and, rarely, jaw necrosis.

Despite improving therapies for androgen-independent prostate cancer, most patients with this disease eventually die as a result of the cancer, often in 12–24 months. Treatment with high-dose steroids can sometimes provide useful palliation. The palliative care of these patients requires a supportive and caring team approach involving the family physician, the urologist, an experienced palliative care team and, of course, the patient's close relatives and friends.

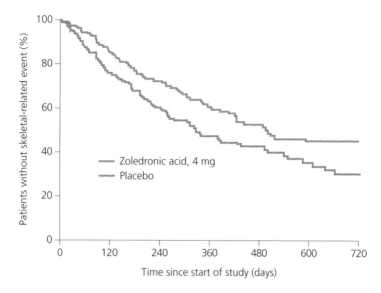

Figure 8.4 Kaplan–Meier estimates of event rates for time to the first skeletal-related event for patients with metastatic prostate cancer randomized to receive zoledronic acid or placebo. Adapted from Saad et al. 2003.

Key points – management of androgen-independent disease

- After an initial response to androgen ablation, the serum PSA value starts to rise as a result of androgen-insensitive cell clones.
- As an initial maneuver, withdraw any antiandrogen the patient is taking.
- Introducing low-dose estrogen (such as stilbestrol, 1–3 mg/day) plus aspirin may result in a PSA response, but carries a risk of cardiovascular and thromboembolic complications.
- Treatment with chemotherapeutic agents has, historically, been disappointing, but docetaxel has been shown to improve survival and quality of life.
- The bisphosphonate zoledronic acid has been reported to delay significantly the occurrence of skeletal events in patients with metastatic prostate cancer.

Key references

Beer TM, Eilers KM, Garzotto M et al. Weekly high-dose calcitriol and docetaxel in metastatic androgen-independent prostate cancer. *J Clin Oncol* 2003;21:123–8.

Beer TM, Pierce WC, Lowe BA, Henner WD. Phase II study of weekly docetaxel in symptomatic androgen-independent prostate cancer. *Ann Oncol* 2001;12:1273–9.

Berry W, Dakhil S, Gregurich MA, Asmar L. Phase II trial of single-agent weekly docetaxel in hormone-refractory, symptomatic, metastatic carcinoma of the prostate. *Semin Oncol* 2001;28(suppl 15):8–15.

Berry W, Dakhil S, Modiano M et al. Phase III study of mitoxantrone plus low dose prednisone versus low dose prednisone alone in patients with asymptomatic hormone refractory prostate cancer. *J Urol* 2002;168:2439–43.

Ellerhorst JA, Tu SM, Amato RJ et al. Phase II trial of alternating weekly chemohormonal therapy for patients with androgen-independent prostate cancer. *Clin Cancer Res* 1997;3:2371–6.

Figg WD, Arlen P, Gulley J et al. A randomized phase II trial of docetaxel (Taxotere) plus thalidomide in androgen-independent prostate cancer. *Semin Oncol* 2001;28(4 suppl 15):62–6.

Friedland D, Cohen J, Miller R Jr et al. A phase II trial of docetaxel (Taxotere) in hormone-refractory prostate cancer: correlation of antitumor effect to phosphorylation of Bcl-2. *Semin Oncol* 1999;26 (suppl 17):19–23.

Kantoff PW, Halabi S, Conaway M et al. Hydrocortisone with or without mitoxantrone in men with hormone-refractory prostate cancer: results of the cancer and leukemia group B 9182 study. *J Clin Oncol* 1999; 17:2506–13.

Kish JA, Bukkapatnam R, Palazzo F. The treatment challenge of hormone-refractory prostate cancer. *Cancer Control* 2001;8:487–95.

Lewington V, McEwan AJ, Ackery DM et al. A prospective, randomized double-blind crossover study to examine the efficacy of strontium-89 in pain palliation in patients with advanced prostate cancer metastatic to bone. *Eur J Cancer* 1991;27:954–8.

Logothetis CJ. Docetaxel in the integrated management of prostate cancer. Current applications and future promise. *Oncology* 2002; 16(suppl 6):63–72.

Petrylak DP, Tangen CM, Hussain MH et al. Docetaxel and estramustine compared with mitoxantrone and prednisone for advanced refractory prostate cancer. *N Engl J Med* 2004;351:1513–20.

Picus J, Schultz M. Docetaxel (Taxotere) as monotherapy in the treatment of hormone-refractory prostate cancer: preliminary results. *Semin Oncol* 1999;26(suppl 17): 14–18.

Saad F, Gleason DM, Murray R et al. A randomized, placebo-controlled trial of zoledronic acid in patients with hormone-refractory metastatic prostate carcinoma. *J Natl Cancer Inst* 2002;94:1458–68.

Saad F, Gleason DM, Murray R et al. Zoledronic acid is well tolerated for up to 24 months and significantly reduces skeletal complications in patients with advanced prostate cancer metastatic to bone. Presented to American Urological Association, 26 April – 1 May 2003. *Proc Am Urol Assoc* 2003;abstract 1472.

Savarese DM, Halabi S, Hars V et al. Phase II study of docetaxel, estramustine, and low-dose hydrocortisone in men with hormone-refractory prostate cancer. A final report of Cancer and Leukemia Group B 9780. *J Clin Oncol* 2001;19:2509–16.

Scher HI, Kelly WK. Flutamide withdrawal syndrome: its impact on clinical trials in hormone-refractory prostate cancer. *J Clin Oncol* 1993;11:1566–72.

Small EJ, Baron A, Bok R. Simultaneous antiandrogen withdrawal and treatment with ketoconazole and hydrocortisone in patients with advanced prostate carcinoma. *Cancer* 1997;80:1755–9.

Smith PH, Suciu S, Robinson MR et al. A comparison of the effect of diethylstilbestrol with estramustine phosphate in the treatment of advanced prostatic cancer: final analysis of a phase III trial of the European Organization for Research on Treatment of Cancer. *J Urol* 1986;136:619–23.

Sweeney CJ, Monaco FJ, Jung SH et al. A phase II Hoosier Oncology Group study of vinorelbine and estramustine phosphate in hormone-refractory prostate cancer. *Ann Oncol* 2002;13:435–40.

Tannock IF, Osoba D, Stockler MR et al. Chemotherapy with mitoxantrone plus prednisone or prednisone alone for symptomatic hormone-resistant prostate cancer: a Canadian randomized trial with palliative end points. *J Clin Oncol* 1996;14:1756–64.

Tannock IF, de Wit R, Berry WR et al. Docetaxel plus prednisone or mitoxantrone plus prednisone for advanced prostate cancer. *N Engl J Med* 2004;351:1502–12.

Treatments for prostate cancer can result in a number of complications. Effective management of these will improve the quality of life of affected men.

Sexual function

A diagnosis of prostate cancer alone may be enough to disturb sex lives that, in the age group usually affected, are often already beginning to wane. In one survey, a surprising number of couples erroneously believed that prostate cancer could be transmitted sexually; they therefore voluntarily abstained from sex.

Erectile dysfunction. Treatment of localized prostate cancer often results in sexual dysfunction. Erectile dysfunction is the most common complaint and can occur after all treatments. Improvements in techniques for radical prostatectomy and nerve sparing, such as the use of robotic assistance, have resulted in very significant improvements in this area; however, erectile dysfunction can occur following even the most expert surgery. Unfortunately, it is also sometimes necessary to deliberately resect the cavernous nerves in order to resect widely to avoid positive surgical margins. This, too, can have detrimental effects on erectile function.

Limited success regarding erectile function has been reported for the replacement of resected nerves with sural nerve grafts after surgery (Figure 9.1).

Intracorporeal fibrosis results from the release of transforming growth factor-α (TGFα). As TGFα is released in response to anoxia, therapies that bring oxygenated arterial blood into the corpora and induce erection inhibit its release and may help maintain smooth muscle function. Early administration of pharmaceutical treatments for erectile dysfunction soon after surgery has been shown to improve the time and quality of subsequent erections. Montorsi et al. have shown in a randomized trial that early intracavernosal injections with alprostadil,

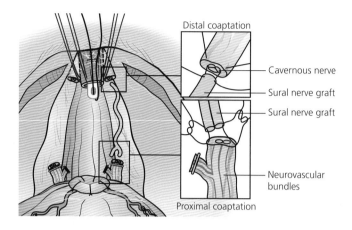

Figure 9.1 Sural nerve graft interposition to restore erectile function following prostatectomy.

once or twice a week, result in early recovery of spontaneous erections after nerve-sparing radical prostatectomy. Early administration of phosphodiesterase type 5 (PDE5) inhibitors daily has also been shown to improve the time and quality of spontaneous erections after bilateral nerve-sparing surgery. Patients refractory to intracavernosal and oral PDE5 inhibitor treatment have the option of using a vacuum constriction device to obtain erections or surgery to insert an inflatable penile prosthesis (Figure 9.2).

External-beam radiotherapy and brachytherapy are both associated with an incidence of delayed-onset erectile dysfunction of 30% or more. Cryotherapy very often results in erectile dysfunction because the neurovascular bundles are included in the freezing zone. Treatment is along the same lines as that for erectile dysfunction following prostatectomy.

Ejaculatory problems. Men undergoing treatment for localized prostate cancer by radical prostatectomy or TURP may also experience ejaculatory problems, though sensation of orgasm is usually preserved. In the case of TURP, semen is still produced, but passes retrogradely

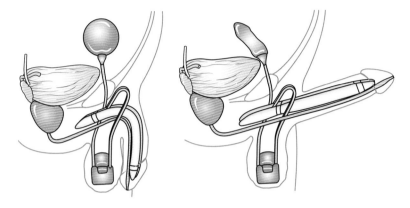

Figure 9.2 An inflatable penile prosthesis.

into the bladder. After radical prostatectomy, in which the entire prostate and seminal vesicles have been removed, no semen is produced, but most patients are still able to achieve orgasm. Patients must be informed about these consequences before surgery. Drugs such as the α_1-blocker tamsulosin, used to treat bladder outflow obstruction, may also cause retrograde ejaculation, but this is reversible on cessation of treatment.

Loss of libido is a common complaint of patients with prostate cancer. It may result from the disease itself causing debilitation or depression. More commonly, it is a side effect of hormone ablation therapy. Bilateral orchidectomy or therapy with LHRH analogs or pure LHRH antagonists is almost invariably associated with loss of libido, as well as erectile dysfunction. Therapy with an antiandrogen can effectively deprive prostate cancer cells of androgen stimulation without such a profound effect on libido or erectile function.

Preservation of sexual function. If this is an important factor in terms of the quality of life of an individual prostate cancer sufferer, then treatment with an antiandrogen as monotherapy may well be considered as an alternative to bilateral orchidectomy or an LHRH analog.

107

Counseling. The most important conclusion to be drawn is that patients with prostate cancer, as well as their partners, should be counseled not only about probable outcomes, but also about the likely effect of the disease and its therapy on their sex lives. A more open and informed approach to this important aspect of prostate cancer would do much not only to counter the anxiety and loss of self-esteem that so often accompany the diagnosis of this frequently encountered malignancy, but also to restore effective sexual function after treatment and thereby maintain an important aspect of quality of life.

Urinary and bowel symptoms

Incontinence following radical prostatectomy. Radical prostatectomy involves removing the prostate gland and some of the bladder neck. The contribution of the bladder neck and prostatic smooth muscle to normal continence is lost following surgery. Operative injury to the remaining rhabdosphincter or its nerve supply is probably the most common factor in post-prostatectomy incontinence. Other factors that may contribute are bladder instability which may have existed before surgery or developed after, and a poorly compliant bladder. Following removal of the urethral catheter after surgery, some degree of immediate stress incontinence is expected, followed by gradual improvement in urinary control. Factors that contribute to the early recovery of continence are:

- younger age of the patient
- experienced surgeon
- bilateral nerve-sparing surgery
- absence of anastamotic stricture.

Performing pelvic floor exercises before and following surgery also helps.

Treatment is initially conservative, with control of fluid intake and pelvic floor exercises. Treatment of bladder instability involves anticholinergic medication. If this fails, options include injection of peri-urethral bulking agent, which has approximately 40% success in the short term. Other options are the insertion of a bulbo-urethral sling or artificial urinary sphincter.

Urinary and bowel symptoms from radiotherapy. During the delivery of radiotherapy, irritative symptoms of urgency and frequency are very common, being considerably worse with HDR brachytherapy and seed brachytherapy than with external-beam radiotherapy. They tend to settle with time, however. Later urinary symptoms can comprise irritative symptoms such as urgency and frequency, pain and even incontinence and can be due to instability, poor compliance, urethral stricture, overflow incontinence, bladder ulcer or a combination of these.

Rectal symptoms may also be troublesome after radiotherapy. Diarrhea, tenesmus and rectal bleeding may all occur. These tend to resolve over time, but patients should be made aware that external-beam radiotherapy is associated with an increased risk of colorectal cancer. Persistent rectal bleeding should be investigated by colonoscopy.

Treatment is also initially conservative, and involves changes to lifestyle as well as identification of the cause and individualized treatment.

Bone health and hormonal therapy

Loss of bone mineral density with androgen-deprivation therapy for prostate cancer is well recognized, with significant loss of bone mineral density occurring within 12 months of starting therapy: the annual loss is approximately 2–8% per year at the lumbar spine and 2–6% at the hip. The loss appears to continue indefinitely while treatment continues, and there is no recovery after therapy is ceased. Just under 20% of men surviving at least 5 years after a diagnosis of prostate cancer have a fracture if treated with androgen-deprivation therapy compared with 12.6% of men not receiving this therapy; this is equivalent to one additional fracture for every 28 men treated with androgen-deprivation therapy.

Vitamin D deficiency exacerbates the development of osteoporosis, so vitamin D status should be evaluated before commencing androgen-deprivation therapy in men with prostate cancer.

Bisphosphonates (zoledronate, pamidronate and alendronate) in men treated with androgen-deprivation therapy have been shown to prevent bone loss in prospective studies and to increase bone mineral density in one randomized controlled trial; bisphosphonates have also been shown to reduce the incidence of skeletal-related events in men with prostate cancer. Further prospective trials are required to assess the efficacy and cost-effectiveness of bisphosphonates in men with prostate cancer who require androgen-deprivation therapy. Until the results from these trials become available, suggestions for the management of bone effects in men on androgen-deprivation therapy include baseline and yearly measurements of bone mineral density. Baseline calcium, phosphate, liver function, thyroid function, 25-hydroxy vitamin D and parathyroid hormone assays should be performed, and calcium and vitamin D supplementation as well as isometric exercises, should be encouraged. Osteonecrosis of the mandible is a rare complication of bisphosphonate therapy.

Key points – management of treatment complications

- Sexual dysfunction is a common sequelae of prostate cancer treatment.
- The implications should be discussed with the patient and his partner.
- Osteoporosis and fracture are common side effects of long-term androgen-deprivation therapy.
- Erectile dysfunction can often be improved with phosphodiesterase type 5 inhibitors, prostaglandin suppositories or injections, or mechanical vacuum devices.
- Loss of libido can be reduced by using antiandrogens as opposed to bilateral orchidectomy or an LHRH analog to treat prostate cancer.

Key references

Ayyathurai R, Manoharan M, Nieder AM, Kava B, Soloway MS. Factors affecting erectile function after radical retropubic prostatectomy: results from 1620 consecutive patients. *BJU Int* 2008;101:833–6.

Carson CC, Burnett AL, Levine LA, Nehra A. The efficacy of sildenafil citrate (Viagra) in clinical populations: an update. *Urology* 2002;60(suppl 2):12–27.

Goldstein I, Lue TF, Padma-Nathan H. Oral sildenafil in the treatment of erectile dysfunction. *N Engl J Med* 1998;338:1397–404.

Holmes-Walker DJ, Woo H et al. Maintaining bone health in patients with prostate cancer. *Med J Aust* 2006;184:176–9.

Kim ED, Nath R, Slawin KM et al. Bilateral nerve grafting during radical retropubic prostatectomy: extended follow-up. *Urology* 2001;58:983–7.

Kirby RS, Watson A, Newling DWW. Prostate cancer and sexual function. *Prostate Cancer Prostatic Dis* 1998;1:179–84.

Montorsi F, Guazzoni G, Strambi LF et al. Recovery of spontaneous erectile function after nerve-sparing radical retropubic prostatectomy with and without early intracavernous injections of alprostadil: results of a prospective, randomized trial. *J Urol* 1997;158:1408–10.

Montorsi F, Nathan HP, McCullough A et al. Tadalafil in the treatment of erectile dysfunction following bilateral nerve sparing radical retropubic prostatectomy: a randomized, double-blind, placebo controlled trial. *J Urol* 2004;172: 1036–41.

Padma-Nathan H, Hellstrom WJ, Kaiser FF et al. Treatment of men with erectile dysfunction with transurethral alprostadil Medicated Urethral System for Erection (MUSE). *N Engl J Med* 1997; 336:1–7.

Padma-Nathan H, McMurray JG, Pullman WE et al. On-demand IC351 (Cialis) enhances erectile function in patients with erectile dysfunction. *Int J Impot Res* 2001;13:2–9.

Paige NM, Hays RD, Litwin MS et al. Improvement in emotional well-being and relationships of users of sildenafil. *J Urol* 2001;166:1774–8.

Penson DF, McLerran D, Feng Z et al. 5-year urinary and sexual outcomes after radical prostatectomy: results from the Prostate Cancer Outcomes Study. *J Urol* 2008;179(Suppl):S40–4.

Saad F, Adachi JD, Brown JP, Canning LA et al. Cancer treatment-induced bone loss in breast and prostate cancer. *J Clin Oncol* 2008;26:5465–76.

Walsh PC, Lepor H, Eggleston JC. Radical prostatectomy with preservation of sexual function: anatomical and pathological considerations. *Prostate* 1983;4: 473–85.

Willke RJ, Glick HA, McCarron TJ et al. Quality of life effects of alprostadil therapy for erectile dysfunction. *J Urol* 1997;157: 2124–8.

Zelefsky MJ, McKee AB, Lee H, Leibel SA. Efficacy of oral sildenafil in patients with erectile dysfunction after radiotherapy for carcinoma of the prostate. *Urology* 1999;53: 775–8.

Prostate cancer has, until recently, been under-researched when compared with other common neoplasms such as breast or colorectal cancers. Perhaps because of increased public awareness of the potentially devastating effects of prostatic malignancy, this balance is now being redressed. It seems probable that increasing awareness and redoubled research endeavors into prostate cancer will eventually translate into improved survival prospects and a better quality of life for the many sufferers of this very prevalent disease.

Chemoprevention

Prostate cancer is, theoretically, a preventable disease (Figure 10.1). Already the finasteride trial has demonstrated that it is possible to

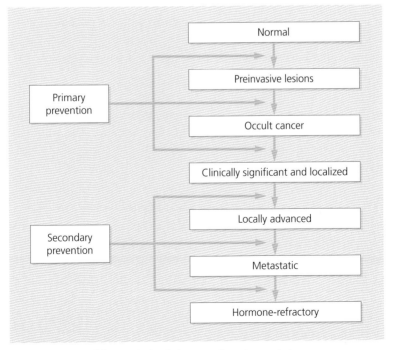

Figure 10.1 Possible prophylactic interventions in prostate cancer.

reduce the incidence of prostate cancer by 24% when finasteride is taken. Dutasteride, a dual 5α-reductase inhibitor, has been evaluated in the REDUCE study; a risk reduction of 23% has been reported, with no increase in the incidence of poorly differentiated tumors. Another trial which could, potentially, have shown an effect for chemoprevention is the SELECT trial. Designed to examine whether supplemental vitamin E and/or selenium reduces the incidence of prostate cancer, the trial was terminated early because of disappointing results.

Earlier detection

The PSA test by itself is clearly inadequate to detect prostate cancer. While measuring free and complexed PSA improves accuracy slightly, major advances in diagnosis have not been made. Further improvements to the diagnosis of early prostate cancer are likely to involve detecting abnormal genes or RNA in the serum or urine. One particular test showing promise is the *PCA3* test. This test detects the mRNA in voided urine of the *PCA3* gene (Figure 10.2), which is highly overexpressed in prostate cancer. The levels are then compared with PSA mRNA in the urine. At a sensitivity of 50%, this test has a specificity of 76%, which is substantially better than PSA. Furthermore, there are indications that *PCA3* may be of value in discriminating between aggressive and more indolent forms of prostate cancer. *PCA3* mRNA levels are independent of PSA and prostate volume, and the combination of *PCA3*, PSA, DRE and prostate volume significantly predicts the likelihood of prostate cancer. Further trials in large populations are required to determine its true usefulness and place.

Other approaches to early detection include profiling protein patterns in the serum by proteomics. Characteristic patterns of proteins in the serum can be diagnostic of prostate cancer and further work is being performed to determine the accuracy of the method. It seems probable that new tests, or variations of existing ones, will continue to improve the ability of clinicians to distinguish early prostate cancer from benign prostatic conditions. Further improvements in diagnosis will result from better identification of men at risk from overexpression of genes such as *LMKT2* and *MSMB*. A possible future approach to screening is shown in Figure 10.3.

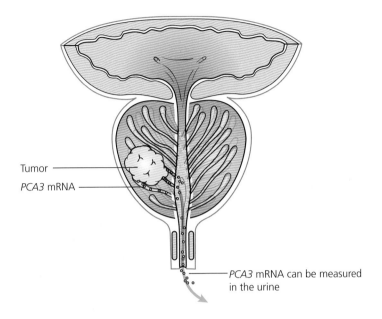

Tumor
PCA3 mRNA

PCA3 mRNA can be measured
in the urine

Figure 10.2 *PCA3* mRNA is detected in the urine, and then related to levels of PSA mRNA.

Better staging and prognostic indicators

One of the problems with current management strategies is the inaccuracy of current staging methods. Improved imaging with, for example, TRUS microbubble technology and MRI with gadolinium enhancement, iron filings or spectroscopy may improve matters. Although earlier detection of prostate cancer will undoubtedly improve the curability of the disease, it also raises the questions of whether a given lesion in an individual patient will or will not progress. Molecular prognostic indicators, such as E-cadherin, anti-cathepsin B and the polycomb group protein EZH2, are currently the subject of intense research, and it seems likely that it will soon be possible to predict more accurately the future behavior of individual prostate cancers. This should facilitate decisions about competing treatment options. Already some predictive markers such as the interleukin-6 receptor and TGFβ

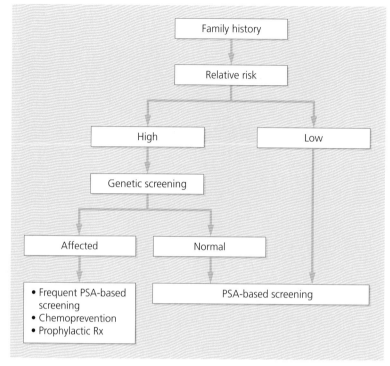

Figure 10.3 A possible scheme for prostate cancer screening in the future.

are being incorporated into nomograms to predict likely outcomes for men with prostate cancer. Detection of circulating prostate cancer cells by polymerase chain reaction has been another avenue of investigation for identifying men likely to have microscopic metastatic disease.

Imaging using monoclonal antibodies against prostate-cancer-specific antigens such as prostate-specific-membrane antigen has been another area of investigation. This method has the advantage of specifically imaging cancer cells. Although results to date have been mixed, further studies are ongoing and it is hoped that the technique will become more accurate as antibodies and target identification improve.

New therapies

For localized prostate cancer, the dominant role of radical prostatectomy and external-beam radiotherapy seems likely to be challenged eventually by newer technologies aimed at ablating the tumor in situ, while minimizing the risks of incontinence and erectile dysfunction. Cryosurgery, HIFU and brachytherapy have already been mentioned in this context, and other modalities such as photodynamic therapy and prostatic hyperthermia are currently being developed.

Laparoscopic techniques. Radical prostatectomy itself may be enhanced by laparoscopic techniques and robotic assistance. Currently, the results with these techniques seem equivalent to those of the open operation, but with technological advances they are likely to become better.

Hormonal manipulation with LHRH analogs seems likely to remain the mainstay of therapy for locally advanced or metastatic disease, though LHRH antagonists and new antiandrogens are currently being evaluated, with preliminary results looking promising. As antiandrogens are refined, they seem likely to be employed increasingly in earlier stages of the disease, when tumor cell sensitivity to androgen withdrawal may be most pronounced.

Currently, the main problems with hormonal therapy for prostate cancer are that 10–20% of patients demonstrate hormonal resistance from the time of initiation of therapy, and the remainder eventually develop androgen independence after an average 36-month initial response period. Better understanding of the mechanisms by which cells acquire resistance to androgen-deprivation treatment is likely to facilitate methods of either delaying or preventing what is currently often an event of ominous prognosis.

A number of novel strategies aim to downregulate pathways active in developing hormonal resistance (Table 10.1). These include inhibitors of tyrosine kinases and antibody inhibitors for growth factor receptors such as epidermal growth factor receptor (EGFR), platelet-derived growth factor receptor (PDGFR) and human epidermal growth factor receptor 2 (HER2). Other approaches include targeting dysregulated factors that allow cancer growth, such as mammalian target of rapamycin (mTOR) or the endothelin axis. The selective endothelin-A-receptor antagonist atrasentan has been reported to delay time to progression in androgen-independent disease, and other new molecules in this class are showing exciting results. For example, overall survival

TABLE 10.1

Novel biological agents in development for treatment of advanced prostate cancer (possibly in combination with chemotherapy)

- Thalidomide
- Lenalidomide (Revlimid)
- High-dose calcitriol
- Imatinib (Gleevac/Glivac)
- Bortezomib (Velcade)
- Bevacizumab (Avastin)
- Proapoptotic agents (e.g. BCL2 antisense oligonucleotide)
- CCI-779 (rapamycin ester) and other inhibitors of mTOR and of AKT
- Lapatinib (Tykerb) and other EGFR, PDGFR, HER2/HER3 inhibitors
- Bisphosphonates
- Atrasenten (Xinlay)
- ZD4054
- Vaccine strategies

AKT, serine/threonine-specific kinase; EGFR, epidermal growth factor receptor; HER, human epidermal growth factor receptor; mTOR, mammalian target of rapamycin; PDGFR, platelet-derived growth factor receptor.

was markedly improved with ZD4054, a specific endothelin-A-receptor antagonist, in a Phase II, placebo-controlled trial involving pain-free or mildly symptomatic men with androgen-independent prostate cancer and bone metastases. A number of these agents have also been tested in combination with docetaxel, which has been shown to be effective in androgen-independent prostate cancer. Further studies on new chemotherapy drugs are also continuing, with satraplatin and epothilones showing promising activity. The cytochrome P450 inhibitor abiraterone has been the focus of much interest recently. However, as yet, relatively few patients have been treated and the drug is not licensed for clinical use.

Vaccines. Anti-prostate-cancer vaccines are also now a not-too-distant prospect. Introducing cytokine genes, such as those encoding interleukin-2 or granulocyte-macrophage colony-stimulating factor (GM-CSF), into harvested prostate cancer cells and subsequently reintroducing them into the host has been shown to enhance local and systemic immunologic antitumor responses. Dendritic-cell-based therapy is also being investigated. In a large trial of men randomized to treatment with a vaccine called sipuleucel-T (Provenge), which contains dendritic cells exposed to modified prostate cancer antigens, or placebo, those treated with the vaccine had a survival benefit of 4.1 months, with minimal side effects. Further studies of vaccine therapy are ongoing.

Gene therapy. The recent spectacular advances in molecular biology have made the prospect of gene therapy an imminent reality. Gene therapy for prostate cancer is likely to proceed down several avenues, including:
- reasserting control over disturbed cell division mechanisms
- introducing cytotoxic agents specifically into prostate cancer cells, leaving normal cells unaffected.

Prostate cancer develops as a result of stepwise activation of oncogenes and deletion of tumor suppression genes. Potentially, oncogenes could be neutralized or deleted, or tumor suppressor genes reinserted by any of the vector methods currently in development.

Concluding thoughts

The prospects for significant advances in the struggle against prostate cancer in the near future are good. The death rate is already beginning to fall, though the decline is happening more rapidly in the USA than in the UK. To earlier diagnosis, better staging, and more effective and less toxic therapy may be added the possibility of effective chemoprevention. Perhaps in the future it may even be possible to identify the 10% of men congenitally at risk of eventually developing clinical prostate cancer by genetic profiling, and thereby target chemoprevention and close surveillance strategies specifically to them. Whatever the future holds, the battle to reduce the morbidity and mortality of prostate cancer seems set to intensify well into the new millennium; family physicians now need to close ranks with urologists and oncologists and strive to ensure that eventual victory is achieved.

Key references

Andriole G. Further analyses from the REDUCE prostate cancer risk reduction trial. *Late-Breaking Abstract 1*. Presented at the American Urological Association (AUA) Annual Meeting, 25–30 April 2009, Chicago, IL, USA.

Anon. A randomized, double-blind, placebo-controlled, multi-center, phase III trial of sipuleucel-T in men with metastatic, androgen independent prostatic adenocarcinoma (AIPC). Presented at the AUA Late-Breaking Science Forum, American Urological Association (AUA) Annual Meeting, 25–30 April 2009, Chicago, IL, USA.

Attard G, Ried AH, Yap TA et al. Phase 1 clinical trial of a selective inhibitor of CYP17, abiraterone acetate, confirms that castration-resistant prostate cancer commonly remains hormone driven. *J Clin Oncol* 2008;26:4563–71.

Bruno RD, Njar VC. Targeting cytochrome P450 enzymes: a new approach in anti-cancer drug development. *Bioorg Med Chem* 2007;15:5047–60.

Chu D, Wu S. Novel therapies in genitourinary cancer: an update. *J Hematol Oncol* 2008;1:11.

Deras IL, Aubin SM, Blase A et al. PCA3: a molecular urine assay for predicting prostate biopsy outcome. *J Urol* 2008;179:1587–92.

Eccles SA, Welch DR. Metastasis: recent discoveries and novel treatment strategies. *Lancet* 2007;369:1742–57.

Gomella L. Chemoprevention using dutasteride: the REDUCE trial. *Curr Opin Urol* 2005;15:29–32.

James ND, Caty A, Borre M et al. Safety and efficacy of the specific endothelin-A receptor antagonist ZD4054 in patients with hormone-resistant prostate cancer and bone metastases who were pain free or mildly symptomatic: a double-blind, placebo-controlled, randomised, phase 2 trial. *Eur Urol* 2008. Epub ahead of print.

Heinonen OP, Albanes D, Virtamo J et al. Prostate cancer and supplementation with alpha-tocopherol and beta-carotene: incidence and mortality in a controlled trial. *J Natl Cancer Inst* 1998;90:440–6.

Lippman SM, Klein EA, Goodman PJ et al. Effect of selenium and vitamin E on risk of prostate cancer and other cancers: the Selenium and Vitamin E Cancer Prevention Trial (SELECT). *JAMA* 2009;310:39–51.

Morris MJ, Scher HI. Novel therapies for the treatment of prostate cancer: current clinical trials and development strategies. *Surg Oncol* 2002;11:13–23.

Nelson PS, Gleason TP, Brawer MK. Chemoprevention for prostatic intraepithelial neoplasia. *Eur Urol* 1996;30:269–78.

Nelson JB, Udan MS, Guruli G, Pflug BR. Endothelin-1 inhibits apoptosis in prostate cancer. *Neoplasia* 2005;7:631–7.

Reid AH, Attard G, Barrie E, de Bono JS. CYP17 inhibition as a hormonal strategy for prostate cancer. *Nat Clin Pract Urol* 2008;5:610–20.

Sanda MG, Ayyagari SR, Jattee EM et al. Demonstration of a rational strategy for human prostate cancer gene therapy. *J Urol* 1994;151: 622–8.

Small EJ, Bok R, Reese DM et al. Docetaxel, estramustine, plus trastuzumab in patients with metastatic androgen-independent prostate cancer. *Semin Oncol* 2001;28(suppl 15):71–6.

Small EJ, Fratesi P, Reese DM et al. Immunotherapy of hormone-refractory prostate cancer with antigen-loaded dendritic cells. *J Clin Oncol* 2000;18:3894–903.

Small EJ, Schellhammer PF, Higano CS et al. Placebo-controlled phase III trial of immunologic therapy with sipuleucel-T (APC8015) in patients with metastatic, asymptomatic hormone refractory prostate cancer. *J Clin Oncol* 2006;24:3089–94.

Thompson I, Goodman PJ, Tangen CM et al. The influence of finasteride on the development of prostate cancer. *N Engl J Med* 2003;349: 215–24.

Valone FH, Small E, MacKenzie M et al. Dendritic cell-based treatment of cancer: closing in on a cellular therapy. *Cancer J* 2001;7(suppl 2): S53–61.

Varambally S, Dhanasekaran SM, Zhou M et al. The polycomb group protein EZH2 is involved in progression of prostate cancer. *Nature* 2002;419:624–9.

Useful resources

UK

Macmillan Cancer Support
89 Albert Embankment
London SE1 7UQ
CancerLine: 0808 808 2020
Nurse information line: 0808
800 1234
www.macmillan.org.uk
www.cancerbackup.org.uk

The Men's Health Forum
32–36 Loman Street
London SE1 0EH
Tel: +44 (0)20 7922 7908
www.menshealthforum.org.uk

The Prostate Cancer Charity
First Floor, Cambridge House
100 Cambridge Grove
Hammersmith, London W6 0LE
Tel: +44 (0)20 8222 7622
Helpline: 0800 074 8383
www.prostate-cancer.org.uk

Prostate UK
6 Crescent Stables
139 Upper Richmond Road
London SW15 2TN
Tel: +44 (0)20 8788 7720
www.prostateuk.org

Prostate Cancer Research Foundation
156 Blackfriars Road
London SE1 8EN
Tel: +44 (0)20 7953 7178
www.thepcrf.org.uk

USA

American Cancer Society
Tel: +1 800 227 2345
www.cancer.org

American Urological Association
1000 Corporate Boulevard
Linthicum, MD 21090
Tel: +1 410 689 3700
www.auanet.org

National Cancer Institute
6116 Executive Boulevard
Room 3036A, Bethesda
MD 20892-8322
Toll-free: +1 800 422 6237
www.cancer.gov/cancertopics/
types/prostate

ZERO The Project to End Prostate Cancer
10 G Street NE
Suite 601 Washington, DC 20002
Tel: +1 202 463 9455
Toll-free: 1 888 245 9455
www.zerocancer.org

Prostate Conditions Education Council
7009 South Potomac St, Suite 125
Centennial, CO 80112
Tel: +1 303 316 4685
Toll-free: 1 866 477 6788
www.pcaw.com

Prostate Cancer Foundation
1250 Fourth Street
Santa Monica, CA 90401
Tel: +1 800 757 CURE (2873)
Main: +1 310 570 4700
www.prostatecancerfoundation.org

Prostate Cancer Research Institute
5777 West Century Boulevard
Suite 800, Los Angeles, CA 90045
Tel: +1 310 743 2116
Helpline: +1 310 743 2110
www.prostate-cancer.org

International
Prostate Cancer Foundation of Australia
PO Box 1332
Lane Cove NSW 1595, Australia
Tel: +61 (0)2 9438 7000
Toll-free: 1800 220 099
www.prostate.org.au

Prostate Cancer Canada
145 Front Street East, Suite 306
Toronto, ON M5A 1E3, Canada
Tel: +1 416 441 2131
Toll-free: 1 888 255 0333
www.prostatecancer.ca

Other useful websites
Johns Hopkins Medicine
James Buchanan Brady Urological Institute
http://urology.jhu.edu

Cancer Research UK
www.cancerresearchuk.org

Embarrassing Problems
www.embarrassingproblems.com

Hormone-Refractory Prostate Cancer
www.hrpca.org

Patient UK www.patient.co.uk

Memorial Sloan-Kettering Cancer Center www.mskcc.org

Mayo Clinic prostate cancer
www.mayoclinic.com/health/
prostate-cancer/DS00043

William Catalona (developer of the PSA test) www.drcatalona.com

Index